How Do We Want to Live?

Gerhard Gründer

How Do We Want to Live?

We Decide Ourselves About Our Future

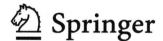

Springer

Gerhard Gründer
Mind and Brain Institute GmbH
Zornheim, Rheinland-Pfalz, Germany

ISBN 978-3-662-64224-5   ISBN 978-3-662-64225-2   (eBook)
https://doi.org/10.1007/978-3-662-64225-2

"For the next two generations: Leonhard, Nikolaj, Philipp, Johann, Finja, and Enjo."

Foreword

From the very beginning of my medical studies, I knew that I wanted to become a brain researcher. The brain was the most complex and difficult organ to understand, but it was also by far the most fascinating. It was a mystery to me how anyone could be interested in such mundane organs as the liver, the prostate, or even the heart. However, the more I became involved with the various aspects of neuroscience—for example, during my practical year in neurology—the clearer it became to me that dealing with diseases of the brain and nerves would not be enough. To this day, what interests me most are the questions about the basis and origins of mind, psyche, and consciousness. So I decided to become a psychiatrist, and I have not regretted it to this day. No medical field is as diverse and multifaceted as this one, and while on the one hand you deal with the basic questions of being human, on the other hand you have to deal with suffering people every single day, to whom you have to offer comfort and help. This is a fascinating and inspiring field of tension that maintains and promotes alertness and creativity.

My first academic teacher was a renowned "biological psychiatrist" and psychopharmacologist, and I owe my path to an academic career to him. In the course of years of clinical and scientific work, I thus also acquired a certain competence in psychopharmacology. Interfering with brain chemistry through chemical substances is an exciting field. The possibilities it has opened up for the treatment of severe mental disorders are impressive, but there is no doubt that poorly conducted pharmacotherapy can also do harm. For decades now, I have also been concerned with the question of how these substances exert their effects. Closely related to this is the question of how the activity of nerve cells gives rise to psychological experience or even an awareness of oneself.

However, I have always been skeptical of ideas that one only has to intervene specifically enough in the brain chemistry to ultimately stop any mental suffering, and people who were completely convinced—not convincing—that it was only a matter of time until we knew enough about the brain to banish psychiatric illnesses from the world astounded me. For me, the experience of self has remained a mystery, and our failure to understand how it arises fills me with humility.

Now I have the feeling that the voices (scientists, brain researchers, but above all psychiatrists) who consider the human being to be a complex biomachine that only needs to be understood well enough to eliminate depression and anxiety are becoming louder and more dominant. Psychological experience is here only an epiphenomenon of biological function. People like to compare the brain to a computer, and artificial intelligence is soon to be able to simulate brain function so well that a mental disorder can be detected before it arises, and if it does, the computer will help us cure it with molecular precision by analyzing all our "biomarkers." The projection goes so far that an Israeli historian tells us that the intervention in our brain is the path to "global happiness."

Is this just a competition of ideas, a discourse among scientists? I am convinced that there is much more at stake here. It is about a dominant, very reductionist worldview that determines how we think about ourselves and that permeates our culture. Our worldviews, however, determine how we live with each other, how we work, how we educate ourselves, and what kind of healthcare system we want. We have accumulated an enormous amount of knowledge about how our genes and our biology determine our thoughts, feelings, and actions. However, we tend to forget the enormous room for maneuver we have. Happiness is not created in the individual brain, but in the social interaction between people. And how we—actively and consciously—shape these interactions will determine our future.

Zornheim, Germany   June 2020
Gerhard Gründer

Contents

Part I

How I Do Not Want to Live

1

Why This Book?

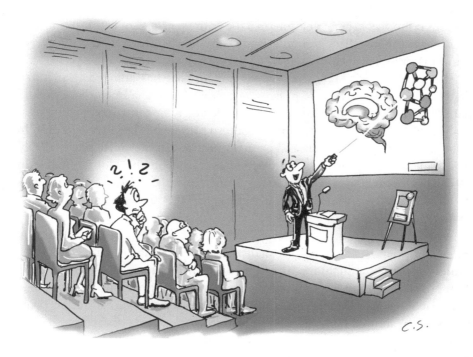

Abstract What motivated the author to write the book? American scientists want to solve the "opioid crisis" in the US through a better understanding of brain chemistry, in the New York Times a columnist celebrates a new drug as the "solution" to rising suicide rates, and a bestselling Israeli author declares intervention in brain chemistry as the path to "global happiness." A biological

© Springer-Verlag GmbH Germany, part of Springer Nature 2022
G. Gründer, *How Do We Want to Live?*, https://doi.org/10.1007/978-3-662-64225-2_1

reductionism is spreading, and a humanistic view of humanity is being called "outdated" by journalists. Are we on the right track?

On a Sunday morning in December 2018, I sat with several hundred other scientists in a packed auditorium at a large conference hotel on the east coast of Florida. The day before, the annual American College of Neuropsychopharmacology (ACNP) convention, held in the first half of December, had begun. At this meeting, which usually takes place in a sunny, warm place in the USA, scientists, mostly from the USA, a smaller part also from other continents, mostly Europe, meet to exchange the latest scientific findings for four and a half days. I myself have been travelling to the USA regularly for many years at the beginning of December to inform myself at this conference about the latest insights in the fields of neurobiology of psychiatric diseases and psychopharmacology. The first morning is usually devoted to large plenary sessions on topics of general interest to the entire participant community. This year it was the so-called "opioid crisis" in the USA: "The opioid crisis: What solutions can science contribute?"

The "opioid crisis" refers to a development that has afflicted the United States in particular over the past two decades. Since the late 1990s, opioid painkillers have been prescribed in the USA largely uncontrolled and increasingly also for mild pain conditions. As a result, there has been an explosion in the number of opiate addicts and opiate overdoses. In the entire year of 1999, less than 1000 people died from opiate overdoses in the United States. In 2017, not even 20 years later, that number of opiate overdose deaths was counted every two weeks! That added up to 28,000 deaths after overdose in 2017!

What did the scientists have to offer at the conference? Here, six top American scientists stepped up to present their solutions to the assembled professional public, including the director of the National Institute on Drug Abuse (NIDA). They spoke about the neurobiology of pain, opiate receptors, pharmacology and biomarkers. Only the first speaker, who introduced the symposium, showed a few numbers illustrating the drama of the opioid crisis before quickly pointing out how "basic knowledge of how the brain works and is affected by drugs, pain, and addiction [...] is necessary for future transformative solutions." None of them talked about possible social or societal causes of the problem, none about possible flaws in the American health care system. Now, one might object that this is a congress for psychopharmacologists, not social scientists, and if one wanted to debate social scientific approaches to solving the crisis, one could go to a congress on social medicine.

But that is not the case. There were a lot of psychiatrists here (including me), including some who treat patients. And in the title of the symposium, "solutions" were offered. How could anyone—and here the word is very apt—be so limited as to believe that the problem of one thousand people losing their lives to opiate overdose every two weeks in the US could be solved primarily by pharmacology and brain chemistry? I have long disagreed with the reductionist models that "biological psychiatry" has to offer as solutions to the enormous disease burden that psychiatric illness has created worldwide. But what was offered here was either incredibly brazen or just naive.

Three months after the symposium in Florida, on March 7, 2019, the New York Times headlined: "Deaths from drugs and suicide reach a record in the US" [1]. The statement was based on 2017 figures. "More than 150,000 Americans died from alcohol- and drug-related deaths and suicide in 2017. Nearly one-third—47,173—were suicides." Those numbers were double what they were in 1999, the year when this type of mortality data began to be collected. The article quotes Benjamin Miller, chief policy officer of the American Well Being Trust: "There are two crises in America right now, one in health care and one in society." The Well Being Trust, according to its website, is a "national foundation dedicated to advancing the mental, social and spiritual health of the nation." According to Miller, feelings of despair, loneliness and lack of belonging contribute to suicides among Americans. An article in the New York Times, published a week before the symposium at the ACNP convention, on November 30, 2018, also states that, "The trend most likely has social causes—lack of access to mental health care, economic stress, loneliness and despair, the opioid epidemic, and the unique difficulties facing small-town America. These are serious problems that require long-term solutions." In the meantime, however, psychiatry desperately needs new treatments, and the author concludes (and this is in the title to his article!), "Ketamine may be the solution" [2]. Ketamine is a drug that has been known for many decades, used in the context of anesthesia and as an analgesic. It was first reported 20 years ago that the substance also had a very rapid—within hours—onset antidepressant effect. Numerous studies conducted since then have confirmed this finding. Then, in 2019, both the U.S. and European health authorities approved a derivative of ketamine, esketamine, for the treatment of treatment-resistant depression (depression is considered "treatment-resistant" when it has not improved on various antidepressants). After many years of virtually no new psychiatric drugs being approved, the approval of esketamine represents a small step forward. But a "solution" to the rising suicide numbers in the US? That strikes me as naive as saying we can reduce the number of deaths from opiate overdose by better understanding the opiate receptor. When, at a press conference held at the end of November 2018 on the occasion of the annual congress of the German Society for Psychiatry and Psychotherapy, Psychosomatics and Neuroscience (DGPPN) in Berlin, I criticized the biological reductionism expressed in such simple notions, a journalist reproached me with an "outdated humanism" in a commentary that appeared a few days later [3].

I have been scientifically involved in psychopharmacology for 30 years. I try to understand how psychotropic drugs work, I try to conduct a therapy with psychotropic drugs that is as rational and scientifically sound as possible, and I have probably treated several thousand patients with antidepressants, antipsychotics, tranquilizers and several other compounds from other classes of drugs. I have also tested new drugs, for and with the pharmaceutical industry, with whom I have often worked closely, advised and from whom I have received fees for lectures. I have often been attacked for this. But I have always kept a critical distance from what I do, and it would never have occurred to me to regard psychiatric drugs as the "solution" to any psychiatric illness. Psychotropic drugs are very beneficial for many patients, they often enable them to live in the community again after only a few days or weeks of treatment. Anyone who has spent a few days in a sheltered ward of a psychiatric hospital cannot seriously doubt that these drugs can be extremely helpful, especially in acute and severe illnesses—acute schizophrenia, for example. People who yesterday were tormented by hearing voices and delusions of persecution state the day after tomorrow that they have been relieved, sometimes even freed, from these modes of experience by drug therapy. And a great many people benefit from long-term therapy with these drugs. But this is about more, this is about worldviews that are behind these "solution approaches".

In fact, most of academic, university psychiatry, not only in the Western world, believes that psychiatric disorders are due to biochemical dysfunctions in the brains of those affected. These molecular dysfunctions, in turn, can be traced back to specific risk genes for the particular disorder. So, in order to successfully treat these diseases, all I have to do is correct the dysfunction as accurately as possible with a drug, and since the dysfunction naturally returns when the drug is discontinued, I have to continue the drug therapy permanently. Of course, it is recognized that to a greater or lesser degree environmental factors and life events also play a role in the genesis of psychiatric illness, more so in one person and less so in another. Ultimately, however, the environment in this model is viewed only as a moderator of the genetic-biological risk for the disorder. These ideas may indeed be true in some severe, strongly genetically determined cases of disease. However, in the vast majority of people who develop psychiatric illness, no biological abnormalities are found. Now it is perfectly legitimate to assume that it is only a matter of time before psychiatry has accumulated enough knowledge to be able to understand the biology of psychiatric illness to a completely different extent than we are currently able to. Biological psychiatrists like to draw the comparison to oncology, which has made enormous progress in recent years. Today, it is often possible to characterise tumours genetically with such precision that it is possible to tailor therapy to the individual patient. The fact that these possibilities have not yet been developed in psychiatry is due to the enormous complexity of the brain. However, in the age of artificial intelligence and "big data", it is finally foreseeable that it will also be possible to treat people with psychiatric diseases with very individual, "personalised" biological therapies, which will mostly be drugs.

However, it goes further than that. We have evolved into a society that pathologizes any psychological discomfort, sadness, and anxiety and declares it a disease. Many negative emotions, however, make perfect sense; they have ensured man's survival in evolution. And even today, they signal to us that something is "wrong." This may be due to us as individuals (and thus indeed to our biochemistry), but it may just as well be due to our environment, our living conditions, the way we work, live, interact with each other. Biological reductionism, as expressed in scientific symposia such as the one I described or even in the newspaper article I quoted, completely ignores this. The Israeli historian Yuval Harari takes this to the extreme in his book "Homo deus" [4]. Harari actually claims here in all seriousness that the improvement of man's living conditions is a model of yesterday. Today, and even more so tomorrow, "global happiness" will be generated by intervening in the biochemistry of the brain. The book has been bought by millions and critically acclaimed. I am sure that most of Harari's readers are not even aware of the worldview being painted here. It is worldviews, buildings of ideas, that determine how we shape our world. I will show in this book that the "homo deus" is a naive and false ideal that is not only unattainable. To aspire to it would also mean ceding man's ability to shape his future to a technocratic elite with their machines. Is that really what we want?

I chose the title of the book so ambitiously because I actually believe that we ourselves decide what image of the world we form. World views, systems of ideas, decide how we as humans want to live in the future. Each individual human being can significantly influence his or her individual destiny; they are not victims of some genetic or otherwise biological program that unfolds by fate. But even more so, we decide how we will live together as a human community in the future. This decision will determine whether we need to inject ourselves with opiates, or any other more sophisticated substances in the future, in order to eliminate feelings of unwillingness or other negative emotions.

I wrote this book as a plea for a humane psychiatry, and such a humane psychiatry is also a political psychiatry. It advocates an improvement in living conditions for as many people as possible, living conditions in which each individual can develop to the best of his or her ability. And it is a plea for a new humanism.

References

1. New York Times (March 7th 2019) Deaths from drugs and suicide reach a record in the U.S. New York Times. https://www.nytimes.com/2019/03/07/us/deaths-drugs-suicide-record.html. Accessed on February 29th 2020

2. New York Times (November 30th 2018) Can we stop suicides? New York Times. https://www.nytimes.com/2018/11/30/opinion/sunday/suicide-ketamine-depression.html. Accessed on February 29th 2020

3. Esanum (November 30th 2018) Wie das menschliche Gehirn, nur besser: Künstliche Intelligenz. Esanum. https://www.esanum.de/today/posts/wie-das-menschliche-gehirn-nur-besser-kuenstliche-intelligenz. Accessed on Febraury 29th 2020

4. Harari YN (2018) Homo deus. Beck, München

2

Taking Stock: Our World at the Beginning of the Twenty-First Century

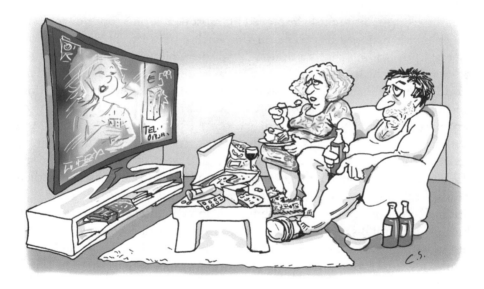

Abstract For most people, life on this earth has become better just in the last 200 years. We live significantly longer, fewer and fewer people are starving or illiterate. However, this development is in marked contrast to our mental health. The global burden of disease from mental disorders is steadily increasing, with more than one billion people affected by a mental disorder or addiction. Depression and stress-associated disorders are particularly common, suicide rates are rising, particularly in the US, and here especially—most worryingly— among young girls. Do we have the right answers to these developments?

© Springer-Verlag GmbH Germany, part of Springer Nature 2022
G. Gründer, *How Do We Want to Live?*, https://doi.org/10.1007/978-3-662-64225-2_2

Contrary to a widespread opinion, living conditions on this earth have improved in many respects for many people over the last hundred years. This is shown by the Swedish scientist Hans Rosling, who died in 2017, in his world bestseller "Factfulness" with many examples and impressive figures to prove it [1]. For example, while in 1800 only about 10% of people were able to read and write, in 2016 it was 86%. While only 65% of girls worldwide were enrolled in school as recently as 1970, this figure was 90% in 2015. As recently as 1980, only 58% of the world's population had access to water from a protected source, but by 2015 the figure had risen to 88%. Whereas in 1970, 28% of the world's population was undernourished (meaning that just 50 years ago, almost one in three people was still suffering from hunger), today that figure is just 11%. In 1950, 28% of children between the ages of 5 and 14 worked full time; in 2012, that figure was 10%. Even if these sober figures conceal the fact that even today too many people suffer from very poor living conditions, it can be seen from an infinite number of other parameters that these have continuously improved for most people and continue to do so, and the vast majority of people on this earth participate in these developments. Thus Rosling paints a thoroughly positive picture of the development of human society. In the introduction to his book he writes: "Think about the world: Wars, violent crime, natural disasters, man-made disasters, corruption. Terrible things are happening, and it feels like everything is only getting worse, right? The rich are getting richer, and the poor are getting poorer. And the numbers of poor people keep increasing. And soon we will run out of resources unless we do something about it, and we do it now. At least that's the picture most people in the West see in the media and carry around in their heads. I call this the over-dramatized worldview. It is incriminating and misleading" [1]. Rosling, together with his son and daughter-in-law, had made it his mission until his death to change this "overdramatized worldview," and he did so with great commitment, not only with his successful book, but also in numerous, internationally acclaimed lectures that took him as far as the World Economic Forum in Davos.

Medical care in most parts of the world has also improved significantly. In every country in the world, life expectancy has increased dramatically over the last century. Across all countries, the average life expectancy today is 72 years. In 1800, it was an unimaginable 31 years for us today! Even in the poorest countries of the world, almost all of which are in Africa, life expectancy is now over 50 years. The countries with the lowest life expectancy are the two African states of Central African Republic and Lesotho, where life expectancy is 51 years. But even there, health care has improved so significantly that people there are now living much older than they were just a few decades ago. In

1800, a today unfathomable 44% of children did not live to see their fifth birthday; today that figure is 4%. In 1980, only 22% of one-year-old children had received at least one vaccination; in 2016, 88% had. Because of the worldwide vaccination campaign of the World Health Organization (WHO), smallpox has been considered eradicated since 1979; in 1850, the disease was still registered in 148 (of 194) countries of the world. While infection with the HI virus (commonly known as the AIDS virus) was still considered a death sentence in the 1980s, today newly infected people have an almost normal life expectancy, and the number of new infections has more than halved in the last 20 years. Today, if a child under the age of 20 develops cancer, there is an 80% chance that this child will survive for at least the next five years. In 1975, this figure was only 58% [1]. Cancer medicine in particular has made enormous progress in recent decades in terms of diagnostics and therapy. If these developments continue, cancer will probably lose its horror completely in the next 20 years. The successes of cancer medicine are only most obvious in the popular press; many other physical diseases can be treated better today than they were just a few decades ago. Popular science literature in particular celebrates the successes of modern biomedicine: "From Silicon Valley comes the next revolution that will radically change our lives: the reinvention of medicine. Tech giants like Google and Microsoft, as well as countless start-ups, are developing data-based computer medicine that is perfectly tailored to individual patients. Already, new diagnostic capabilities are making it possible to detect changes in the body before they become diseases. Spectacular new therapies and highly effective drugs promise to soon give us healthier, significantly longer lives" [2].

However, these positive developments are in striking contrast to our mental health. In October 2018, an international group of scientists, the Lancet Commission on Global Mental Health, presented their report on the state of mental health in the global population. The summary is sobering: "Despite substantial research advances showing what can be done to prevent and treat mental disorders and to promote mental health, translation into realworld effects has been painfully slow. The global burden of disease attributable to mental disorders has risen in all countries in the context of major demographic, environmental, and sociopolitical transitions. Human rights violations and abuses persist in many countries, with large numbers of people locked away in mental institutions or prisons, or living on the streets, often without legal protection. The quality of mental health services is routinely worse than the quality of those for physical health. Government investment and development assistance for mental health remain pitifully small. Collective failure to respond to this global health crisis results in monumental loss of human capabilities and avoidable suffering" [3]. In 1993, the World Bank introduced the concept of "disability-adjusted life years (DALYs)" to measure and standardize the importance of a disease or group of diseases to a society. DALYs combine the number of years of life lost to premature death with the number of years spent with disease-related disability. In 1991, psychiatric disorders accounted for 6.6% of all DALYs worldwide. Since then, their importance in the global burden of disease has steadily increased. In 2016, 9.4% of all DALYs were attributable to psychiatric conditions. This increased much more slowly in richer regions of the world (from 13.6% in 1991 to 16.2% in 2016) than in very poor regions, where—from a low baseline—their importance virtually doubled (from 2.2% to 4.3%). The authors estimate that 13 million deaths were directly or indirectly attributable to psychiatric disorders in 2010 [3], and there is no end in sight to this trend. 800,000 people worldwide take their own lives every year! The economic consequences of this "Mental Health Crisis"—according to the Lancet Commission—are also enormous. It estimates the costs caused by mental illness to be 16 trillion US dollars by 2030. In a press statement given by the lead author of the Lancet report after its release, he said, "The situation is extremely bleak." He said the burden of mental illness had increased "dramatically" worldwide over the past 25 years, partly due to ageing societies and more children surviving into adolescence, yet "no country is investing enough" to address the problem. Further, he said, "No other aspect of health has been more neglected in human history than mental health" [4]. The WHO supports this account by stating that on average across all countries in the world, less than 2% of health system expenditure is spent on mental illness.

According to current figures from the World Health Organization (WHO) in December 2019, based on the Lancet report, 264 million people are affected by depression alone, with older figures suggesting more than 300 million sufferers. Depression currently accounts for the third largest burden of disease worldwide—after back pain and headaches—(measured by days burdened by each condition), but it will have moved up to first place by 2030, according to WHO estimates. WHO writes on its website: "The burden of depression and other mental illnesses is increasing worldwide" [5]. In addition to the enormously high number of people suffering from depression, there are 45 million people affected by dementia, 20 million people suffering from schizophrenia and 45 million suffering from bipolar disorder (formerly manic-depressive illness). The most common mental illness, however, which often remains unmentioned in statistics, is the group of anxiety disorders, which, according to the current figures of the WHO, affect 284 million people. In total, the number of people affected by mental illnesses amounts to

970 million—almost one billion! This does not even take into account addictions (now called "substance use disorders"), which affect a further 175 million people worldwide, including 107 million people with alcohol dependence. Each year, more than 300,000 babies are born with what is called fetal alcohol syndrome. These children start life with a significant handicap due to developmental delays caused by their mother's alcohol consumption during pregnancy. In 2017, the year the Lancet Report figures were collected, there were 7.55 billion people living on Earth. Of these, if you include addictions, more than 1.1 billion people were affected by a mental illness, which was almost one in seven people!

In recent years, the major health insurers have repeatedly examined the mental health of the German population in various studies. For its "Stress Study 2016", published by the Techniker Krankenkasse (TK) under the title "Entspann Dich, Deutschland" (English: "Relax, Germany"), the opinion research institute Forsa surveyed 1200 German speakers in June and July 2016 on their stress levels and relaxation strategies in everyday life, leisure and work [6]. 23% of respondents, who represented a representative cross-section of the population, said they were often stressed, and a further 38% sometimes, making a total of 61% of adults in Germany. In their 2013 study, the figures had been 20% and 37% respectively. The proportion of those who were stressed at least sometimes was particularly high in the age groups 30 to 39 (82%) and 50 to 59 (76%). It is only after the age of 60 that the proportion of people who feel stressed decreases significantly.

Employment appears to have a significant influence on the experience of stress. While only 45% of those not in gainful employment suffer from stress at least sometimes, 77% of full-time and 63% of part-time employees feel stressed. Interestingly, the perception of stress increases with the level of education and with the disposable monthly income. I will return to the significance of our work, and especially how we work, for our well-being in the last part of the book.

For many years, the statistics of all health insurance companies have shown that the personal perception of stress and mental health go hand in hand. According to the Health Report 2018 of the one of the large German health insurance funds (DAK), the days of incapacity to work per 100 insured persons due to mental illness increased from 76.7 days to 249.9 days from 1997 to 2017, which is more than a threefold increase. The number of incapacity days increased from 2.5 to 7.0 per 100 insured persons. While the days and cases of incapacity for work for most somatic illnesses have been at a relatively constant level for years and have even been falling for individual types of illness, they are rising steadily for mental illnesses, with no end to this trend in sight. In 2017, mental illnesses accounted for 16.7% of all days lost by DAK policyholders. Behind diseases of the musculoskeletal system—these are primarily diseases of the spine—they are in second place in the total volume of days lost [7]. Among women, mental illnesses are even ahead of musculoskeletal disorders in terms of the volume of days lost from work. Women are more affected by mental illnesses than men over the entire life span. At least this is the case if one measures the extent of the illness in terms of diagnosis or incapacity to work statistics. If we look at the suicide statistics, a different picture emerges (see also Chap. 3): men take their own lives much more frequently than women, which is certainly also due to the fact that they seek professional help much less frequently than women and therefore do not appear in many health insurers' statistics. In both sexes, the number of days of incapacity to work increases steadily with age. For women over 60, their volume is four times as high as for young people between 15 and 19, and for men almost six times as high [7].

Within the group of psychiatric disorders, by far the most frequent causes of incapacity to work are depression, followed by the so-called "reactions to severe stress and adjustment disorders", which, like depression, must be regarded as often stress-associated.

The TK (TK is another large German health insurance funds) Stress Study 2016 highlights the digitalisation of society as a key determinant of the increasing experience of stress. Many people feel that the working world in particular is becoming faster and faster and that they can no longer cope with the demands. The study shows a clear correlation between the frequency of digital media use and the personal experience of stress. Although this does not prove causality, it is noticeable that people who are rarely or never stressed use digital media significantly less than those who are frequently stressed [6]. Interestingly, academic psychiatry around the world has hopes that digitalization will solve not only diagnostic problems (how do we diagnose mental illness more reliably and earlier?) but also therapeutic problems (how do we treat mental illness more successfully and, above all, more sustainably?) in a very fundamental way. Physicians such as the American cardiologist Eric Topol even go so far as to claim that the widespread application of artificial intelligence in medicine will lead to healthcare becoming more human again ("How artificial intelligence can make healthcare human again" [8]). I will return to this in Chap. 4.

Remarkably, the high activity of adolescents on social media is also blamed with the rising suicide rate among adolescents in the US for years, especially among girls. While this was only 1.7 per 100,000 for girls in 1999, it had significantly more than doubled to 4.2 suicides by 2017. For boys, it rose, less sharply, from 4.9 to 8.7 suicides per 100,000 people [9]. What is of particular concern to American researchers is that the increase in the suicide rate among American girls is accelerating exponentially. Until 2014, it had been increasing at about 3% per year, but since then it has been increasing at 10% per year. As one American suicide researcher summarizes the findings on the causes of this worrying trend, "The data show that girls' social media use is more likely to lead to interpersonal stress. Compared to boys, girls are more likely to use social media, more likely to be exposed to cyberbullying, and cyberbullying is more likely to cause stress and emotional problems in girls than in boys. Social media use is also more likely to cause depression in girls."

Very recent figures from the USA show that the frequency of depression there has increased over the last two decades. Whereas in 2005 6.6% of the population had suffered from depression in the previous 12 months (the so-called 12-month prevalence), by 2015 this figure had risen to 7.3% [10]. However, the prevalence rates among adolescents (12–17 years) and young adults (18–25 years) have risen particularly sharply.

The fact that constant use of mobile phones and tablets also affects student performance was taken into account by the French government in July 2018 by banning the use of these devices in pre-primary, primary and secondary schools, i.e. for all students up to the age of 15. It also aims to reduce bullying via social media [11]. The psychiatrist Manfred Spitzer from Ulm has been warning about the dangers of uncritical digitalisation of school education and its effects on our mental health for years, e.g. for the first time in his book "Digital Dementia" [12] and in the following years in several other books, which were critically received by many specialist colleagues.

Parallel to the epidemic increase of stress-associated diseases, overweight and obesity have been increasing dramatically for decades. Overweight is characterized by a Body Mass Index of 25–30 kg/m^2 (BMI is calculated by dividing body weight in kg by height in m squared; thus, a man of 80 kg and a height of 1.85 m has a BMI of 23.4 kg/m^2), obesity refers to a condition with a BMI greater than 30 kg/m^2. Figures from 2008 for the US show that 35% of adults were affected by obesity, which was 78.6 million people. The resulting cost to the health care system was estimated at $147 billion [13]. The same group of scientists calculated that if the prevalence of overweight and obesity continues to develop as it has over the past 20 years, obesity will affect 51% of Americans as early as 2030. Keeping the prevalence (proportion of people in the total population who have a disease or risk factor at any given time) of obesity at 2010 levels would result in cost savings of a staggering $500 billion [14].

Since 1962, the prevalence of obesity among Americans has almost tripled; in 1962 it was only about 13%. Figures published by the OECD for Europe show that the situation here appears to lag that in the USA by only a few years [15]. In 2012, more than half (53%) of the adult population in Europe were overweight or obese (the man in the above example with a height of 1.85 m would have a BMI of 30 with a body weight of 103 kg, he would then be "obese"). In 2012, more than 50% of adults were overweight or obese in 17 of the EU member states. On average across all EU states, 16.7%, or one in six, were obese, but again there were wide regional variations, with 8% in Romania to over 25% in Hungary and the UK [15]. Ten years earlier, in 2002, the figure had been around 13%. However, in all countries for which figures are available, the prevalence increased between 2002 and 2012, in some cases significantly. Both sexes are equally affected. In some countries, such as Slovenia, Luxembourg or Malta, the proportion of men is significantly higher, in others, such as Latvia or Hungary, the proportion of women.

The most comprehensive set of figures worldwide was published in 2016 in the medical journal *Lancet* [16]. The authors analyzed trends for adults in 200 countries for the period between 1975 and 2014, during which time—across all countries—BMI increased from a mean of 21.7 kg/m² to 24.2 kg/m² for men and from 22.1 kg/m² to 24.4 kg/m² for women. In 2014, the lowest BMI values (21.4 kg/m²) for men were found in Central Africa and South Asia, and the highest (29.2 kg/m²) in Polynesia and Micronesia (that is, the so-called "South Seas"). For women, they ranged from 21.8 kg/m² in South Asia to 32.2 kg/m² in Polynesia and Micronesia. The incidence of under-weight (defined as BMI < 18.5 kg/m²) decreased from 13.8% to 8.8% for men and from 14.6% to 9.7% for women from 1975 to 2014. In 2014, the prevalence of underweight was still very high at 23.4% (men) and 24.0% in South Asia, i.e. particularly in India and its neighbouring countries. During the same period, the prevalence of obesity tripled from 3.2% to 10.8% in men and doubled from 6.4% to 14.9% in women. So while underweight was two to four times more common than obesity in 1975, today more people worldwide are obese than underweight (see also above the figures published by Hans Rosling in his book). In 2014, 5.0% of women (2.3% of men) worldwide were severely obese (defined by a BMI > 35 kg/m²), and the authors of the Lancet study predict that if trends continue, more women will be severely overweight than underweight by 2025 [16].

The incidence of overweight and obesity in children and adolescents is also worrying. It increased in girls from 0.7% in 1975 to 5.6% in 2016, and in boys from 0.9% to 7.8%. This is an eightfold increase in both sexes [17]. As in adults, the prevalence of obesity in 2016 is particularly high in Polynesia and Micronesia, at more than 30%, but also alarming in North Africa, the Middle East, some Caribbean countries, and the United States, at more than 20%. In recent years, however, the prevalences of obesity in children and adolescents have reached a plateau at a high level in many countries, but in other countries, especially in South, Southeast and East Asia, the increase has accelerated [17].

The OECD also notes in its biennial health report that overweight and obesity are more prevalent in socioeconomically disadvantaged populations. This is particularly true for women. Educational attainment and risk of obesity correlate across Europe, again more strongly for women than for men. Factors contributing to the increase in overweight and obesity, particularly in industrialised countries, include the increasing availability of energy-dense foods and widespread lack of exercise. However, financial worries, especially when chronic or recurrent, are also risk factors for overweight and obesity [15]. A large Finnish study that analyzed data from the entire Finnish population over the period between 1996 and 2014 recently found that people with lower socioeconomic status also have a higher risk of being admitted to a hospital for mental illness. As household income increases, the risk steadily decreases. Nevertheless, a decrease in the number of hospital admissions over the 20 years of the observation period was only found in the highest income population group [18]. Do both trends—the increase in overweight and obesity on the one hand and mental illness, especially depression, on the other—possibly represent manifestations of the same cultural aberrations? Australian researchers have recently formulated the hypothesis that the increasing use of antidepressants (I will discuss this in more detail in Chap. 3) and the unbroken trend towards more overweight and obesity may be causally related and follow the same mechanisms. Both trends have now reached pandemic proportions—that is, as we all know since the Corona pandemic, an epidemic that crosses continental boundaries [19]. Obesity is associated with an increase in the risk of numerous diseases, including not only diabetes mellitus and cardiovascular disease, but also cancers or sleep disorders. The risk of depression also increases and, conversely, depression increases the risk of overweight and obesity, but also of many other diseases. A large French/British long-term study over several decades also recently concluded that socioeconomic status in middle age has a very significant influence on the later risk of frailty, disability and multimorbidity [20].

So the question that arises here—and which I want to discuss in this book—is whether we as a society have the right answers to these challenges. Does medicine in particular, and especially modern psychiatry, have the right answers? Living conditions on earth have improved for many people as a result of enormous scientific, medical, and technological developments that have accelerated in recent decades. We are increasingly better able to treat and often even cure physical illnesses, which has led to an enormous extension of our lifespans, especially in the last century. Some psychiatrists and health policy makers never tire of insisting that the incidence of mental illness has not increased. It is just that many people today are more willing to face up to their mental health problems and seek treatment. Moreover, mental illnesses today are diagnosed earlier and better, and often treated more quickly. Critics who point out that the number of prescriptions for antidepressants has been increasing for the past twenty years counter that more of these drugs actually need to be prescribed if all sufferers are to be treated adequately. There is an undersupply of qualified psychiatric therapy. Even if all this is correct, the worldwide burden of disease caused by mental illnesses has, as we have seen above, reached threatening proportions, and if all the forecasts are correct, it will significantly exceed the burden of disease caused by any physical illness in just a few years. At the same time, the statistics of the WHO and other organizations probably underestimate the importance of mental illnesses considerably, because they do not capture their influence on many physical illnesses.

What is definitely expressed in the statistics of health insurers is that many people no longer feel up to today's living conditions. Globalization and the increasing technologization of our everyday life has led to an acceleration of all life processes, which overtaxes the psychological resilience of more and more people. Sleep disorders, fear of the future, stress and burn-out are now part of our daily companions, and everyone knows at least one, often several, sufferers. If we believe the Israeli historian Yuval Noah Harari, whom I mentioned in the opening chapter, the solution to this problem is not to improve people's living conditions—that was yesterday!—but to intervene in human biochemistry. In his world bestseller "Homo deus" Harari argues that, now that man has increased his life expectancy and his power over nature, the next step is to increase "global happiness" . Then the "humanist revolution" would be complete. Harari's vision is only consistent with the approach of modern biomedicine. Psychiatric research, which is strongly dominated by neurobiology, has been trying for decades to better analyze the complicated "human biomachine" at a cost of billions. Mental illness is understood here as a malfunction of the brain, which is to be repaired by means of ever better, more targeted drugs that intervene in the brain. In the future, people should be better adapted to an often stressful and increasingly hostile professional and social environment. Artificial intelligence and the digitalization of medicine are also understood primarily as a means of better understanding humans as complex, deterministic biomedical machines and thus being able to intervene in them in a more targeted manner. I will devote myself to the ideological and scientific foundations of this approach in the following two Chaps. 3 and 4.

In this book I will discuss the question of whether we want to live in a world in the future in which man is adapted to his environment and medicine serves to optimize man, or whether we want to create living conditions in which we become more satisfied and happier people as we are. The Harariian world view of "Homo deus" is contrasted with a world view in which man is neither a victim of his biology nor of his social environment, but an active creator of their interaction with each other. He is an actor in a complex social structure, the rules of which he determines, and thus he decides on the physical and mental health and well-being not only of himself, but of human society. A passive biomechanism, which as an individual increasingly feels itself to be the victim of global trends over which it no longer believes it has any influence and which, in the event of malfunction, must be repaired and optimised by medication, thus becomes an active shaper of the human society of the future.

In Chaps. 5 and 6, I will show that the incidence and significance of many of the major common diseases of the twenty-first century (e.g., overweight and obesity, dementia, and depression) can be significantly reduced by changes in our lifestyle. Exercise, diet, and meditation represent proven measures in numerous studies to change not only a person's physical health, but also their mental health. Through social change, poverty reduction and education alone, vast improvements in the health and quality of life of many people can be achieved.

In Chap. 7 I will again discuss the modern biomedical worldview and its very concrete implications for our physical and mental health. This worldview suggests that we are determined by our genes (and more recently by epigenetic influences, we will return to this later). But this is only half the truth. The "mind" also influences biology, social systems influence the nature of the individuals that compose the system. Man is not only a victim of his biology, he also has a choice as to how he will live in the future. He is the active shaper not only of his environment, but also of the interaction of his biology with that environment.

Finally, in Part 2 of the book, I will outline in six chapters a worldview in which humans actively shape their future and thus create the framework conditions of their physical and mental health. We decide whether to intervene in our biochemistry or to maintain and increase our future well-being by shaping our living environment—the design of workplaces, cities, but above all our education system. We really do have a choice—we are not the determined pawns in the concert of medical and IT conglomerates.

References

1. Rosling H (2018) Factfulness. Wie wir lernen, die Welt so zu sehen, wie sie wirklich ist. Ullstein, Berlin
2. Schulz T (2018) Zukunftsmedizin. Deutsche Verlagsanstalt, München
3. Patel V, Saxena S, Lund C et al (2018) The Lancet Commission on global mental health and sustainable development. Lancet 392:1553–1598
4. Reuters. Mental health crisis could cost the world $16 trillion by 2030. October 10th 2018. https://www.reuters.com/article/us-health-mental-global/mental-health-crisis-could-cost-the-world-16-trillion-by-2030-idUSKCN1 MJ2QN. Accessed on December 19th 2019
5. World Health Organization, WHO. Depression. https://www.who.int/news-room/fact-sheets/detail/depression. Accessed on May 6th 2020
6. Techniker Krankenkasse (2016) Stressreport 2016. https://www.tk.de/resource/blob/2026630/9154e4c71766c410dc859916aa798217/tk-stressstudie-2016-data.pdf. Accessed on May 5th 2020
7. Deutsche Angestellten-Krankenkasse (DAK) (2018) DAK-Gesundheitsreport 2018. https://www.dak.de/dak/download/gesundheitsreport-2018-pdf-20737 02.pdf. Accessed on May 5th 2020
8. Topol E (2019) Deep medicine. Basic Books, New York
9. Yu B, Chen X (2019) Age and Birth Cohort-Adjusted Rates of Suicide Mortality Among US Male and Female Youths Aged 10 to 19 Years From 1999 to 2017. JAMA Netw Open 2(9):e1911383
10. Weinberger AH, Gbedemah M, Martinez AM et al (2018) Trends in depression prevalence in the USA from 2005 to 2015: widening disparities in vulnerable groups. Psychol Med 48:1308–1315
11. Die Zeit (July 30th 2018) Parlament beschließt Handyverbot an Schulen. Die Zeit. https://www.zeit.de/politik/ausland/2018-07/frankreich-parlament-schulen-handyverbot-mobiltelefon. Accessed on December 22nd 2019
12. Spitzer M (2014) Digitale Demenz. Droemer Verlag, München
13. Finkelstein EA, Trogdon JG, Cohen JW, Dietz W (2009) Annual medical spending attributable to obesity: payer-and service-specific estimates. Health Aff (Millwood) 28:w822–w831
14. Finkelstein EA, Khavjou OA, Thompson H et al (2012) Obesity and severe obesity forecasts through 2030. Am J Prev Med 42:563–570
15. OECD (2014) Health at a Glance: Europe 2014. OECD Publishing
16. NCD Risk Factor Collaboration (NCD-RisC) (2016) Trends in adult body-mass index in 200 countries from 1975 to 2014: a pooled analysis of 1698 population-based measurement studies with 19.2 million participants. Lancet 387:1377–1396
17. NCD Risk Factor Collaboration (NCD-RisC) (2017) Worldwide trends in body-mass index, underweight, overweight, and obesity from 1975 to 2016: a pooled analysis of 2416 population-based measurement studies in 128.9 million children, adolescents, and adults. Lancet 390:2627–2642

18. Suokas K, Koivisto AM, Hakulinen C et al (2020) Association of income with the incidence rates of first psychiatric hospital admissions in Finland, 1996-2014. JAMA Psychiatry 77:274–284
19. Lee SH, Paz-Filho G, Mastronardi C et al (2016) Is increased antidepressant exposure a contributory factor to the obesity pandemic? Transl Psychiatry 15(6):e759
20. Dugravot A, Fayosse A, Dumurgier J et al (2020) Social inequalities in multimorbidity, frailty, disability, and transitions to mortality: a 24-yearfollow-up of the Whitehall II cohort study. Lancet Public Health 5:e42–e50

3

The Response of Modern Biomedicine

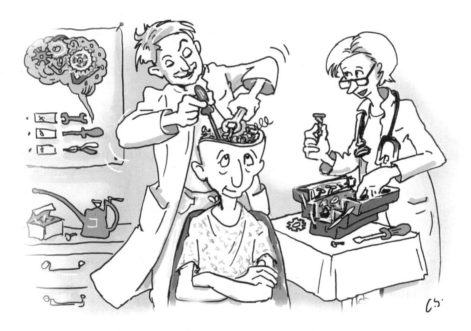

Abstract For more than twenty years, prescriptions of antidepressants have been increasing in all industrialized countries of the world. In Germany, they have more than doubled since 2005. Up to 10% of adults, and in the USA even more than 12%, take an antidepressant on a permanent basis. At the same time, however, we have not become mentally healthier. While psychotropic drugs are a blessing in many severe mental disorders, reducing suffering, the prescription of antidepressants in particular today often represents an inadequate attempt to adapt people to living, housing and working conditions that are experienced as increasingly hostile. They reduce the intensity of feelings such as sadness and fear, which are evolutionarily meaningful because they motivate changes in personality and environment.

We have seen in the second chapter that living conditions for most people almost everywhere on earth have improved significantly during the last 100 years. People today have more to eat, they drink cleaner water, they die less often from infectious diseases, and they are better educated. All of this has led to significant increases in life expectancy around the world, even in the poorest countries. We have also found that this is in striking contrast to people's mental health. The World Health Organization talks of more than 300 million people suffering from depression. There is no sign of this number decreasing; unlike many physical illnesses, mental illnesses are steadily increasing as a percentage of the total global burden of disease. Modern medicine has celebrated significant successes in the twentieth and early twenty-first centuries in the fight against many physical illnesses. Since the middle of the twentieth century, psychiatry has also been trying to transfer the recipes for success of biomedicine to psychiatry. Here we want to analyse what is behind it and what has been achieved? Are we on the right track?

According to the Pharmaceuticals Prescription Report, which analyses the prescriptions of medicines paid for by the statutory health insurance (SHI) in Germany every year, 717 million defined daily doses (DDD) of antidepressants were prescribed in 2005. The value indicates the dose of a drug prescribed in the main indication on average per day. This value more than doubled to 1.515 billion DDD by 2018, i.e. within a decade [1]. Significantly fewer antipsychotics (these are drugs for psychoses, very severe mental illnesses, which also include schizophrenia, for example) were prescribed, although here too the number of prescriptions was increasing (2005: 251 million DDD; 2018: 340 million DDD). The number of prescriptions for tranquilizers actually decreased significantly over the same period (2005: 155 million DDD; 2018: 86 million DDD). However, this is probably at least partly due to the fact that this group of drugs is often prescribed on private prescription. Probably about half of tranquilizer prescriptions therefore do not show up in SHI statistics. What does the figure of 1.5 billion DDD antidepressant prescriptions in Germany mean? In 2018, there were just under 83 million people living in Germany. The number of antidepressants prescribed would have been sufficient to supply all citizens, from newborns to the very old, with an antidepressant for a good 18 days. Or in other words: with this amount, more than four million German citizens could be treated with an antidepressant for the entire year, i.e. all 365 days of the year.

In other countries of the European Community, the situation is comparable, with significant regional differences. According to figures from the Organisation for Economic Co-operation and Development (OECD), the number of antidepressant prescriptions in Europe doubled between 2000 and 2010, with prescriptions of 52 DDD per 1000 European inhabitants in 2010. In 2012, this figure had risen again by a further almost eight percent to 56 DDD [2]. According to the OECD, Germany was slightly below the European average, though the increase from 47 DDD in 2010 to 52 DDD was higher in percentage terms. These figures can also be understood more vividly: About 5% of all people in Europe, from infants to the elderly, take an antidepressant throughout the year. The highest prescription figures for antidepressants are found in Scandinavian countries, led by Iceland (2010: 101 DDD, 2012: 109 DDD), followed by Denmark (2010: 84 DDD, 2012: 83 DDD) and Sweden (2010: 76 DDD, 2012: 81 DDD). Denmark is also the only country in Europe where prescriptions decreased slightly from 2010 to 2012, but also at a very high level. So in Scandinavia, on average, 10% of all citizens take an antidepressant throughout the year! If you are now tempted to assume that these figures reflect the increased incidence of depression associated with less sunshine in the north, you are mistaken. Portugal prescribes as many antidepressants as Denmark (2010: 79 DDD, 2012: 85 DDD). In a European comparison, this puts Portugal in second place. The lowest antidepressant prescription rates are found in Estonia (2010: 16 DDD, 2012: 21 DDD), Hungary (2010: 26 DDD, 2012: 27 DDD) and Slovakia (2010: 29 DDD, 2012: 30 DDD), but in all three countries the rates are increasing [2].

However, these figures are dwarfed by those reported by US health authorities. The U.S. National Center for Health Statistics (NCHS) also analyzes antidepressant prescription figures at regular intervals in their National Health and Nutrition Examination Surveys. The most recent data were reported in August 2017 for the period 2011 to 2014 [3]. Their 2011 report for 2005 to 2008 had stated that antidepressants were the drug class with the third most frequent prescriptions. In the age group of 18 to 44 years, antidepressants had even been prescribed most frequently. Compared to the period 1988–1994, antidepressant prescriptions had increased by 400% by the period 2005–2008 [4]. The trend continued until 2014: Whereas 7.7% (5.1% of men and 10.0% of women) of the U.S. population over 12 years of age had reported taking an antidepressant in the past month in 1999–2002, 12.7% (8.6% of men and 16.5% of women) had done so in 2011–2014, meaning that one in eight

U.S. citizens had taken an antidepressant in the past month. "In the last month" sounds comparatively innocuous in this context. About a quarter of those on antidepressants say they have been taking them for more than 10 years, and another 20% between 5 and 10 years. If we also count people who have been taking antidepressants for between 2 and 5 years as long-term users, then the number of long-term users among the 12.7% of people treated with antidepressants rises to almost 70% [3].

These figures correspond very well with those available for all psychotropic drug groups taken together [5]. According to these figures, 16.7% of all 242 million adult Americans between the ages of 18 and 85 were prescribed a psychotropic drug at least once in 2013, if the three drug groups antidepressants, tranquilizers (anxiolytics, sedatives, hypnotics) and antipsychotics are combined. The figure would be even higher if other groups such as antidementives (drugs for dementia) or stimulants (stimulant drugs given mainly for attention deficit hyperactivity disorder) were also taken into account. Similar to Germany, antidepressants are most commonly prescribed in the United States. 12% of all adult Americans received a prescription for such a drug in 2013. 8.3% received at least one prescription for a tranquilizer and 1.6% for an antipsychotic [5]. Again, these numbers clearly show that the fact that the statistics included all individuals who were prescribed a psychotropic medication only at least once does not mean that these medications are only prescribed on a short-term basis. 84% of those included received at least three prescriptions or had been receiving their medication since 2011 or earlier. On average, those who were prescribed a psychotropic drug on a long-term basis received as many as ten prescriptions a year. It is assumed that in eight out of ten cases, these were permanent therapies [5]. The authors of the study found significant differences in psychotropic drug prescription frequency with respect to ethnicity, age, and gender. While nearly 21% of white Americans were prescribed a psychotropic drug in 2013, this was barely 9% among Latin Americans, and less than 5% among Asians. Five times more whites than Asians were prescribed an antidepressant. Older people were more likely to be prescribed a psychotropic drug than younger people (ages 18–39: 9%; 60–85: 25%), and women more likely than men. In particular, women are prescribed antidepressants significantly more often than men, more than twice as often. The most frequently prescribed psychotropic drugs were the antidepressants sertraline and citalopram, which were prescribed to 6.2 million and 5.4 million Americans respectively (these two drugs are also the most frequently prescribed antidepressants in Germany). Among the ten most frequently prescribed psychotropic drugs were six antidepressants, which were taken by a total of just under 26 million adult Americans. They were prescribed an average of five to six times during the observation year, which means that these figures also indicate that they are predominantly long-term therapies. This further means that more than ten percent of all adult Americans take an antidepressant on a long-term or permanent basis.

Interestingly, the authors found no significant differences in terms of ethnicity, age and gender in the frequency of prescribing antipsychotics. The indication for prescribing these substances is much narrower, and it is usually a consultant psychiatrist who makes the first prescription.

The figures are in astonishing contrast to the suicide rates published by the Centers for Disease Control and Prevention (CDC), the supreme authority for the protection of public health in the USA, at the beginning of June 2018 [6] and which were also reported in the German press. According to this report, suicide rates in the USA rose in all states, with the exception of Nevada, between 1999 and 2016, in some cases drastically. On average, the suicide rate rose by 25% during this period. In 25 states, it increased by more than 30%, with the largest increase in North Dakota at 57%. In 2016, 45,000 people over the age of 10 took their own lives in the United States. Suicide is the tenth leading cause of death there. According to the World Health Organization (WHO), the suicide rate in the USA in 2016 was 15.3 (the suicide rate is given per 100,000 inhabitants). In Germany, according to the WHO, it was not much lower that year, at 13.6 [7]. It is noteworthy that, according to the CDC, more than half of the people who took their own lives did not suffer from a diagnosed psychiatric illness.

In Germany, more than 10,000 people took their own lives in 2015. This means that suicide kills almost three times as many people as road traffic accidents. According to the WHO, the suicide rate worldwide was 10.6 [7]. It is highest in Lithuania (31.9), Russia (31.0) and South Korea (26.9), while the lowest rates are reported for Antigua, Barbados and the Bahamas, where they are below 2.0. Among the G7 countries, Japan has the highest suicide rate at 18.5 and Italy the lowest at 8.2. The median suicide rate in Europe in 2016 was 15.4.

The New York Times headlined "How Suicide Quietly Morphed Into a Public Health Crisis" after the release of the CDC's figures; [8]. It states, "Drugs and psychiatric treatment are more widely available than ever before. Yet suicide rates in the United States are rising". The rising suicide rate, it says, is a serious indictment of the American mental health system. It has been accompanied by a huge increase in the number of Americans diagnosed with depression or anxiety disorder, who are also treated with appropriate medications.

A few weeks earlier, on April 7, 2018, the same newspaper had headlined—this time even on its front page: "Many people taking antidepressants discover they cannot quit" [9]. According to the newspaper's research, more than 15 million adults, or 7% of the U.S. population, have been taking antidepressants for more than five years. That number has nearly doubled since 2010 and more than tripled since 2000, it said. 25 million adults had been taking antidepressants for at least two years, and this number had increased by 60% since 2010 [9]. The New York Times analyzed the figures of the National Health and Nutrition Examination Survey. According to this survey, 13.4 million citizens of the United States had taken antidepressants in 1999/2000. In 2013/2014, that number had risen to 34.4 million, almost a threefold increase. White women over the age of 45 are especially likely to take antidepressants long-term; they account for 58% of people taking these drugs for more than five years, according to the NYT. Older women make up 20% of the total population, but they take more than 40% of all antidepressants, it said.

Remarkably, in almost all countries of the world, suicide rates are significantly higher for men than for women. In the USA and Germany, it is more than three times higher for men than for women. So are the very people who really need drug treatment, namely the group of older men, not getting it? Many psychiatrists believe that the increasing number of prescriptions for antidepressants reflects an undersupply of these drugs to people. The OECD wrote in its 2014 report that the increasing prescription of antidepressants had a variety of reasons. These include, for example, the "greater intensity and duration of treatment"—with all the problems discussed by the New York Times. But also discussed is the expansion of indications to include milder forms of depression, anxiety disorders, or even social phobias. This expansion of the scope of application for antidepressants is to be discussed critically. However, the greater social acceptance of mental disorders and people's willingness to seek help and be treated also play a role [2]. Economic reasons, e.g. economic crises, are also held responsible for the increase in the consumption of antidepressants. The OECD counters that the consumption of antidepressants did increase by 23% between 2007 and 2012, i.e. in times of economic crisis. However, this increase was lower than in the previous five years (2002–2007: 44%). Similar ratios are reported for Portugal (2002–2007: 60% increase; 2007–2012: 30% increase). However, in Germany, which was much less affected by the crisis than most southern European countries, consumption increased much more than there between 2007 and 2012, by 50% [2].

In any case, in its June 8, 2018 coverage of the rising suicide numbers, the New York Times asks the critical question, "If the treatment is so effective, why hasn't its increasing prevalence halted, or even reversed, the rise in suicide rates?" [8]. Thomas Insel, who was director of the U.S. National Institutes of Mental Health (NIMH) from 2002 to 2015 and thus one of the most influential psychiatrists in the world for more than a decade, is quoted by the newspaper as saying, "That's the question I've wrestled with: Are we possibly causing an increase in morbidity and mortality with our interventions?" This is a self-critical and highly significant question for the discipline. Imagine: Here is one of the most important representatives of academic psychiatry asking whether the substances whose mass prescription has been propagated for decades by the authoritative representatives of the discipline, himself included, actually lead to a worsening of the course of the disease! Insel then continues, however, "I don't think so. I think that the need for psychiatric care has increased so much that its expansion has simply not been sufficient so far to have an impact on what is a tremendous social change" [8].

In response to the New York Times article reporting on the difficulties of stopping antidepressant pharmacotherapy, many psychiatrists, especially American psychiatrists, of course, reacted with the usual reflexes. A letter signed by nearly 40 psychiatrists at New York's Columbia University stated, "For practicing psychiatrists and the overwhelming number of patients, withdrawal symptoms are very low on the priority list. […] Although withdrawal syndromes are not particularly well researched, the clinical consensus is that they exist, but that they are rare and always treatable. […] Affective and anxiety disorders are common, debilitating, and often inadequately treated. That a greater proportion of affected Americans are now receiving treatment should be welcomed, not derided" [10].

However, what psychiatrists express here by virtue of their supposed expertise is by no means "clinical consensus". Scientists from the University of Bologna in Italy have systematically analysed the literature on the subject and focused on the group of selective serotonin reuptake inhibitors (SSRIs) [11]. This is the chemical name of the most common group of antidepressants in use worldwide today. They found a surprisingly large number of studies that had systematically examined the question. They conclude that withdrawal syndromes (a syndrome is a complex of symptoms typically occurring together) can occur with any SSRI, but that they are particularly common when paroxetine—a commonly prescribed SSRI—is discontinued. Precise data on the frequency of the occurrence of withdrawal syndromes are difficult to provide, according to this review. Even slow dose reduction does not prevent them, and the data even suggest that slow tapering has no significant advantages over abrupt discontinuation. A withdrawal syndrome typically begins a few days after discontinuation and lasts for a few weeks. However, many deviations from this course are possible, from a delayed onset to a very tardy and prolonged course. In particular, after treatment with paroxetine, withdrawal syndromes lasting up to one year have been documented, and three cases of persistent disorders due to paroxetine withdrawal are found in the literature. Further, these colleagues write, "An editorial published in the late 1990s asserted that antidepressant withdrawal reactions were preventable and easily treated. The evidence we have assembled suggests otherwise". The conclusions from their research are very clear: "The term 'discontinuation syndrome' has steadily replaced 'withdrawal syndrome' in the literature on SSRIs. This change has been strongly supported by the pharmaceutical industry to emphasize that SSRIs do not produce dependence and that these symptoms are substantially different from those seen with benzodiazepines [which are tranquilizers such as Valium]. Clinicians are familiar with the withdrawal phenomena that occur after discontinuing alcohol, benzodiazepines, barbiturates [powerful, addictive sleep aids], opioids [powerful painkillers such as morphine], and stimulants [stimulant drugs such as Ritalin]. The results of this review suggest that they need to add SSRIs to the list of substances that can potentially trigger a withdrawal syndrome. The term discontinuation syndrome' trivializes the potential for harm from SSRIs and should be replaced with 'withdrawal syndrome'" [11].

In a recent online survey, people taking an antidepressant were asked about the occurrence of 20 different side effects and their severity [12]. 1431 people from 38 countries responded. Single withdrawal symptoms were reported by 59% of respondents. Even more common were "feeling emotionally numb" (71%), feeling "foggy or detached" (70%), "feeling not like myself" (68%), "sexual difficulties" (66%), "drowsiness" (63%), and a "reduction in positive feelings" (60%). From this, the authors of the survey concluded that if side effects had been asked directly, there would have been much higher frequencies than had been assumed, especially when it came to emotional, psychological or interpersonal problems. However, it cannot be ruled out that the figures are too high after all, because people suffering from the side effects asked about would certainly have been more likely to respond to the survey than those who were not affected by them.

A particular problem is emotional blunting, which is reported by many people who take antidepressants for a long time. At the University of Oxford, 669 patients taking antidepressants were assessed for signs of emotional blunting using a specially designed questionnaire and compared with 150 people who had recovered from depression and were no longer taking antidepressants

[13]. The researchers found signs of emotional blunting in 46% of patients taking antidepressants, regardless of the type of medication, although this appeared to be slightly—not statistically significantly—less common under one particular antidepressant (bupropion, this drug is not one of the SSRIs discussed above). However, it was also found that emotional blunting was related to the severity of any remaining depressive symptoms. The findings were summarized as follows: "Emotional blunting is reported by nearly half of patients treated with antidepressants. It appears to occur with all monoaminergic antidepressants [almost all antidepressants available today are "monoaminergic", i.e., they affect the metabolism of the monoamines serotonin, norepinephrine, and dopamine]. Emotional blunting, however, is not simply a side effect of antidepressants, but also a symptom of depression" [13].

These data suggest that withdrawal syndromes and serious side effects such as emotional blunting are the rule rather than the exception with long-term treatment with antidepressants. Many psychiatrists underestimate these problems and tend to deliberately downplay them. It should be remembered, however, that antidepressants are potent drugs that have significant effects on the brain. Their prescription has unfortunately reached an unreasonable degree of frivolity today.

What may be experienced as a great relief for people with an acute, possibly severe depression, namely the distance to one's own, then usually tormenting feelings, may become a burden in the long term, especially when the depression has subsided. And it is not only positive emotions whose absence is suddenly perceived as a reduction of vitality. Negative emotions also have their important function for the social interaction of people. They have an evolutionary biological function, they signal to the individual a situation that requires change. The will to change the personal situation—and also the situation of third parties—only arises through negative emotions. What the pharmacological influence of emotions means for the social behavior of humans is little studied and experimentally also poorly accessible. However, impressive findings have been made on this in rats. Researchers at the University of Chicago showed that, with some practice, one rat will release a second rat from a cage [14]. A cage that is empty or filled with inanimate objects will not be opened. When the rat is confronted with two cages, one occupied by a conspecific and the second filled with chocolate, both cages are opened; the rats then share the chocolate with each other. These findings are considered evidence of empathic behavior even in rodents. Other scientists have shown that rats prefer to share their food with other rats rather than eat alone [15]. Now, when rats are treated with the benzodiazepine midazolam, a tranquilizer (or anxiolytic, substances given to quickly relieve anxiety), they show significantly less helping behavior toward their caged conspecific. A cage containing chocolate is also still opened under midazolam [16]. Unfortunately, no studies have examined empathic behavior in rats under antidepressants. However, rats in which the amygdala (the almond nucleus in the temporal lobe of the brain), a central integrating organ for emotions, is damaged also no longer share their food with conspecifics [17]. Reducing the sensitivity of the amygdala to strong, emotion-laden stimuli is considered a possible mechanism of action for antidepressants. It is certainly somewhat speculative now, but could the increasing prevalence of antidepressants in all Western industrial societies lead to the loss of empathic, prosocial behavior?

The fear of former NIMH director Thomas Insel that our pharmacological interventions could trigger an increase in morbidity and mortality is also not as far-fetched as it seems at first glance. In fact, there is quite a bit of evidence, both from animal experiments and from human clinical research, that antidepressant pharmacotherapy may actually worsen the course of depression in some circumstances. Scientists at the University of Modena in Italy induced a depression-like phenotype in mice by exposing them to chronic stress, i.e., behavior and biological changes typically observed in humans suffering from depression [18]. They then treated the animals with either the selective serotonin reuptake inhibitor fluoxetine (the first antidepressant from the SSRI class, which made a worldwide splash as "Prozac", in Germany as "Fluctin"; it was already introduced in the late 1980s) or with a placebo. However, they carried out this treatment under two different environmental conditions: Either the animals were now kept in an environment enriched with pleasant, stimulating environmental stimuli (a so-called "enriched environment"), or they were further stressed. The results of this study are remarkable. The animals treated with fluoxetine in a stimulating environment showed significant improvement in their depression-like phenotype. This improvement was more pronounced than in the animals treated with placebo. However, in the animals that were further stressed, the depression-like phenotype actually increased, and even more so than in the placebo-treated animals. Thus, the antidepressant fluoxetine led to a worsening of the depression-like state here compared to treatment with an ineffective substance. How do the study authors explain these startling findings? They suggest that the SSRI does not lead to an improvement in mood per se, but rather improves transmission between neurons (so-called "neuronal plasticity"), thereby making the animal—and, if the results could be applied to humans, humans as well—more receptive to stimuli from the environment. They conclude that the effects of SSRIs (and possibly antidepressants in general) are not determined by the substance itself, but only induced by it, but ultimately driven by environmental factors. If the stressful environmental factors are not changed, the course of the disease may be worsened by pharmacotherapy [18].

But are these findings transferable to humans? In fact, there are at least indications that they are. The same group of Italian scientists examined the data from a large American study on drug therapy for depression (the so-called STAR*D study: Sequenced Treatment Alternatives to Relieve Depression). They found that in a subpopulation of 600 patients, all of whom had been treated with the SSRI citalopram (probably the most prescribed antidepressant worldwide in the last decade or more), sociodemographic variables significantly influenced treatment outcome. A better response to therapy was found among those with better education, higher income, private health insurance, and those who were employed. This effect was dose-dependent. The dosages of citalopram in depression therapy are usually between 20 mg and 40 mg. The researchers found an effect of patients' socioeconomic circumstances only in patients treated with 40 mg of citalopram; the effect was not significant in the 20 mg group. The influence of socioeconomic circumstances was 37 times stronger in the 40 mg group than in the 20 mg group. The authors conclude from their results that citalopram increases the influence of environmental influences on mood in a dose-dependent manner, in case of doubt then also in a negative sense [19]. It has long been known that socioeconomic conditions have a significant influence on the success of treatment for depression. What is new is the finding that this could be directly related to the dose of the antidepressant administered. Prospective studies will be needed to confirm the link. However, there is further evidence that what psychiatrists call "treatment resistance" may be caused by the (drug) therapy in the first place. A very prestigious group of scientists from Yale University, USA, studied the response of more than 2500 patients treated with one of two different antidepressants or placebo in clinical trials [20]. They described the response to the antidepressant in the different groups by "trajectories", curves representing the severity of their depression over time. Interestingly, patients who had been treated with placebo in the trials studied could be described by a single trajectory. However, patients who had been treated with verum (Latin for "the real thing," meaning an active antidepressant) followed two trajectories. One trajectory described patients who were "responders" to therapy, and the second trajectory described patients who did not respond to therapy (non-responders). Remarkably, the patients who did not respond to antidepressant therapy (which was almost 25% of all patients who received an antidepressant) had a worse outcome than the patients who were treated with placebo [20]. The question that the authors of the article unfortunately do not discuss at all is whether antidepressant pharmacotherapy leads to a worse course of illness in a not insignificant proportion of patients treated with it than if they had not been treated or had only been treated with a placebo. However, the result is important for the interpretation of clinical studies with antidepressants. In such studies, the outcome of patients treated with a verum is averaged and compared with the outcome of patients treated with placebo. However, the worse outcome in antidepressant non-responders compared to the outcome in the placebo group depresses the mean of all patients in the verum group, which may ultimately lead to the modest differences between verum and placebo in antidepressant trials [20]. Just half of all studies comparing an antidepressant to a placebo find superiority of the antidepressant.

Unfortunately, the response to antidepressant pharmacotherapy is also no guarantee that depression will not occur again in the future. This is confirmed by numerous studies on relapse prevention with antidepressants, and the above-mentioned team of researchers from Yale also came to this conclusion. One third of patients whose depression was successfully treated with an antidepressant had a relapse in the following six months [21]. In contrast, when they continued to be treated with a placebo after the acute depression had subsided, 46% of patients relapsed. This is a moderate difference of 13% [21]. Whereas in the past the idea was that an antidepressant would correct a biological "defect", e.g. a deficiency of serotonin, today we must abandon this simplistic notion. The parallel with diabetes mellitus, in which a molecule missing from the organism is supplied from the outside and thus a largely functioning blood sugar regulation is restored, unfortunately fails completely here. Thus, the American researchers conclude, "The protective effect of continued medication is much smaller, only 13%, than one might have expected or hoped for. These findings suggest that strategies for reducing or forestalling the return of depression symptoms need to be developed and widely implemented in depression treatment" [21].

A well-known and increasingly popular method of depression treatment is physical activity and sports. Their positive effect on depression is now undisputed. It becomes interesting when sports and antidepressant pharmacotherapy are compared as treatment options. A group of scientists at the renowned Duke-University in Durham, USA, undertook such a study twenty years ago, which received much attention [22]. 156 elderly patients (all were at least 50 years old) with depression were randomly assigned to three groups. They either underwent a four-month program of aerobic endurance training (30 min three times per week at 70% of maximum heart rate) or received the SSRI antidepressant sertraline. A third group underwent treatment with a combination of the two interventions. After four months, 60% of patients in the exercise group had achieved remission (remission is when the severity of depression, as measured by a scale, has fallen below a certain threshold; depression is then considered to have virtually abated), 66% in the antidepressant group, and 69% in the combination group. These differences were not statistically significant. However, patients treated with sertraline had achieved remission more quickly [22]. Patients were followed up another six months later, for a total of ten months [23]. While two-thirds of the patients in the sports group and in the combination group continued their sports program, just under half in the antidepressant group had also started sports activity. The use of antidepressants also differed significantly between the groups after ten months: 7% of the patients in the sports group had started taking an antidepressant in the meantime. In the combination group, 40% and in the antidepressant group 26% of the patients were still taking such a drug.

Patients who had been treated in the sports group and had thus achieved remission had a sixfold lower risk of relapsing into depression than those who had been treated with sertraline. The difference between the antidepressant group and the combination group was not statistically significant. Only eight percent of patients who had achieved remission with the help of exercise relapsed, but 38% of those who had achieved it on the antidepressant. Interestingly, the relapse rate was not significantly lower in the combination group (31%) than in the antidepressant group, i.e., instead of an additive effect of the two interventions, which might be expected, the administration of the SSRI seemed to prevent the beneficial effects of exercise training [23]. In this regard, the authors write, "Interestingly, combining exercise with medication conferred no additional advantage over either treatment alone. In fact, the opposite was the case, at least with respect to relapse rates for patients who initially responded well to treatment. This was an unexpected finding because it was assumed that combining exercise with medication would have, if anything, an additive effect. The reasons for this are open to speculation" [23].

One reason for this unexpected result could be that patients who were assigned to one of the two groups in which they received sertraline had a certain negative attitude towards pharmacotherapy. In the same vein, it has been suggested that patients who use exercise to free themselves from depression develop a stronger sense of "self-efficacy" than patients taking a drug. While on the one hand, beliefs of the type "I had to work hard at it, but I beat this depression" may have developed, improvement with a medication may promote beliefs such as "I took an antidepressant, and this one helped me out of depression" [23]. In the latter case, the patient does not feel that he has actively overcome his illness, but rather that he has been passively at the mercy of a disturbance in his metabolism that has been corrected by a drug. These are important considerations to which we shall return several times later.

Even though the number of patients in this study was quite small and methodological weaknesses leave room for interpretation, the study as a whole has been received very critically of antidepressants. The question remains why patients who had taken an antidepressant in addition to exercise were more likely to have a disadvantage from the medication.

Psychotropic drugs, including antidepressants, are effective medicines, and for many people with severe mental illness they are a blessing. Nevertheless, the debate about the extent of their effectiveness, or whether they are effective at all, has been going on regularly for decades. Psychotherapeutic procedures are no more effective than pharmacotherapy, and for many patients psychotherapy is not a treatment option. This controversy will not be explored further here, although it has been detailed in this chapter that available medications are far from truly curing mental illness. Anyone who has worked in an acute psychiatric hospital ward knows the impressive treatment results that can be achieved with psychotropic drugs. People who hear haunting voices and suffer from frightening delusions often experience dramatic improvement in their symptoms within days when treated with what is called an antipsychotic (a drug that is effective against psychosis). They return to life in a way that no other form of therapy can achieve. However, these applications of psychotropic drugs are not the issue here.

The question of the extent to which our mental health can be improved by medication touches on much more fundamental issues than how best to treat severe mental illness. It also revolves around the question of whether medicines or chemical "substances" (the term is probably more accurate, because "medicine" or "drug" implies the treatment of a condition) can improve our well-being. The Israeli author Yuval Noah Hariri, who has already been mentioned several times, considers in his world bestseller "Homo deus "the increase of global happiness as one of the three essential tasks of what he calls the "humanist revolution". The "new human agenda" now includes increasing life expectancy ("immortality"), increasing human power ("divinity"), and increasing happiness. He writes, "The second major project on the human agenda will probably be to find the key to happiness. Throughout history, numerous thinkers, prophets, and ordinary people have defined happiness, rather than life itself, as the highest good. [...] In the twentieth century, GDP [gross domestic product] per capita was probably the most important metric for evaluating national success. [...] But thinkers, politicians, and even economists today argue that GDP should be supplemented or even replaced by GHP, Gross Happiness Product" [24] (translated to English from the German translation of the book).

How, if we believe Harari, will happiness be increased? His prescription is simple: "If science is right, and our happiness is determined by our biochemical system, then lasting happiness can be guaranteed simply by influencing that system. Forget economic growth, social reform and political revolutions—to increase global happiness levels, we need to manipulate human biochemistry. We have already begun to do just that in the last few decades. Fifty years ago, psychiatric drugs were heavily stigmatized. Today, that stigma has been broken. In any case, an increasing proportion of the population is taking psychotropic drugs regularly, not only to cure distressing mental illnesses, but even for very mundane depression and occasional moods."

But if it really is the case that "economic growth, social reforms and political revolutions" no longer play a role in the individual perception of happiness, how does Harari explain the fact that Afghanistan, a country whose citizens are permanently threatened by civil war and terror, has by far the highest incidence (22.5% of people are affected by it at any given time) of depression in the world?

Harari describes a worldview that no longer dominates only medical thinking, but also our social system. If a person does not function sufficiently—is not sufficiently "happy"—he is adapted to the system. In case of doubt, this already happens in childhood: "For example, an increasing number of school children are turning to stimulants such as Ritalin. In 2011, 3.5 million American children were given medication for ADHD (attention deficit hyperactivity disorder). In the UK, that number rose from 92,000 in 1997 to 786,000 in 2012. The aim of this had originally been to treat attention deficit disorder, but today even perfectly healthy children take such drugs to boost their performance and meet the growing expectations of teachers and parents. [...] But until now, everyone has agreed on at least one thing: for better education, we need to change schools. Today, for the first time in history, at least some people believe that changing the biochemistry of students would be more effective."

Harari, however, does not realize that it is precisely this attitude, this worldview, that he promotes and praises as humanity's path to the future when he writes: "All this, of course, is not really enough. [...] For that we will have to change our biochemistry and redesign our bodies and minds. So we're working on just that. You can argue whether that's good or bad, but it would seem that the second great project of the twenty-first century—to provide global happiness—is also about remodeling Homo sapiens so that he can feel eternal joy."

Does this remind us of anything? Aldous Huxley described exactly this scenario in his visionary novel "Brave New World", which was already published in 1932! In a world that elevates the stability of society to a maxim, the permanent satisfaction of the citizens' needs is the ultimate goal. This is achieved through unrestrained consumption and sex. Feelings of unwillingness are nipped in the bud by the drug "soma". "Today—this is called progress—our old people work, they copulate, they have and need no time to relax from fun, never idle hours to sit down and think—or, should there be a gap inadvertently in the tightly knit block of their distractions, there is always soma, our delicious soma, a half-gram for the half-holiday, a gram for the weekend, two grams for the trip to the heady East, three for a dark eternity on the moon, so that when you return you always find yourself on the other side of the yawning hole, [...]" [25] (translation to English from the German translation of the novel).

The American cardiologist Eric Topol conjures up a similar scenario in his book "Deep Medicine", in which he praises the blessings of artificial intelligence and "Big Data" for medicine, and he explicitly refers to Harari. Only with Topol, it is not the biochemistry of the individual that is the determinant of happiness, but his "data":

"We are clearly a long, long way from the world Harari describes, if we can even get there. But, like depression, happiness is something we could potentially use to measure and improve. Pascal Budner and colleagues at MIT collected about 17,000 pieces of data, including heart rate, location, and weather conditions via smartwatches in a small study of sixty people over two months. The users entered their state-of-mind data four times a day using a "happimeter", picking from nine emojis. While it's hard to conclude much from the study, it represents one of the first to use AI [artificial intelligence] to understand and track the flip side of depression. Indeed, we are still at the earliest point of defining happiness; we do know what the principal reason for its absence is—mental health disorders" [26].

In the next chapter, let's take a closer look at what artificial intelligence and the digitalization of medicine might mean—all promise aside—for our future as a human society.

References

1. Schwabe U, Paffrath D, Ludwig WD, Klauber J (2019) Arzneiverordnungs-Report 2019. Springer, Berlin
2. OECD. Health at a Glance: Europe 2012 und 2014. OECD Publishing
3. Pratt LA, Brody DJ, Gu Q (2017) Antidepressant use among persons aged 12 and over: United States, 2011–2014. NCHS Data Brief 283:1–8 https://www.cdc.gov/nchs/data/databriefs/db283.pdf. Accessed on May 7th 2020

4. Pratt LA, Brody DJ, Gu Q (2011) Antidepressant use in persons aged 12 and over: United States, 2005–2008. NCHS Data Brief 76:1–8

5. Moore TJ, Mattison DR (2017) Adult utilization of psychiatric drugs and differences by Sex, Age, and Race. JAMA Intern Med 177:274–275

6. Centers for Disease Control and Prevention (CDC) (7. Juni 2018) Suicide rates rising across the U.S. Press release. https://www.cdc.gov/media/releases/2018/p0607-suicide-prevention.html. Accessed on May 7th 2020

7. Weltgesundheitsorganisation (World Health Organization, WHO) (2018) Global Health Observatory Data. Suicide Rates 2016 (per 100000 population) http://wwwwhoint/gho/mental_health/suicide_rates_crude/en/. Accessed on May 14th 2020

8. New York Times (8. Juni 2018) How suicide quietly morphed into a public health crisis. https://www.nytimes.com/2018/06/08/health/suicide-spade-bordain-cdc.html. Accessed on May 7th 2020

9. New York Times (7. Apr. 2018) Many people taking antidepressants discover they cannot quit. https://wwwnytimescom/2018/04/07/health/antidepressants-withdrawal-prozac-cymbaltahtml. Accessed on May 7th 2020

10. New York Times (9. Apr. 2018) Withdrawing from antidepressants. https://wwwnytimescom/2018/04/09/opinion/antidepressantshtml. Accessed on May 7th 2020

11. Fava GA, Gatti A, Belaise C, Guidi J, Offidani E (2015) Withdrawal symptoms after selective serotonin reuptake inhibitor discontinuation: a systematic review. Psychother Psychosom 84:72–81

12. Read J, Williams J (2018) Adverse effects of antidepressants reported by 1,431 people from 38 countries: emotional blunting, suicidality, and withdrawal effects. Curr Drug Saf 13:176–186

13. Goodwin GM, Price J, De Bodinat C, Laredo J (2017) Emotional blunting with antidepressant treatments: a survey among depressed patients. J Affect Disord 221:31–35

14. Ben-Ami Bartal I, Decety J, Mason P (2011) Empathy and pro-social behavior in rats. Science 334:1427–1430

15. Hernandez-Lallement J, van Wingerden M, Marx C et al (2015) Rats prefer mutual rewards in a prosocial choice task. Front Neurosci 8:443

16. Ben-Ami Bartal I, Shan H, Molasky NM et al (2016) Anxiolytic treatment impairs helping behavior in Rats. Front Psychol 7:850

17. Hernandez-Lallement J, van Wingerden M, Schäble S, Kalenscher T (2016) Basolateral amygdala lesions abolish mutual reward preferences in rats. Neurobiol Learn Mem 127:1–9

18. Alboni S, van Dijk RM, Poggini S et al (2017) Fluoxetine effects on molecular, cellular and behavioral endophenotypes of depression are driven by the living environment. Mol Psychiatry 22:552–561

19. Chiarotti F, Viglione A, Giuliani A, Branchi I (2017) Citalopram amplifies the influence of living conditions on mood in depressed patients enrolled in the STAR*D study. Transl Psychiatry 7:e1066
20. Gueorguieva R, Mallinckrodt C, Krystal JH (2011) Trajectories of depression severity in clinical trials of duloxetine: insights into antidepressant and placebo responses. Arch Gen Psychiatry 68:1227–1237
21. Gueorguieva R, Chekroud AM, Krystal JH (2017) Trajectories of relapse in randomised, placebo-controlled trials of treatment discontinuation in major depressive disorder: an individual patient-level data meta-analysis. Lancet Psychiatry 4:230–237
22. Blumenthal JA, Babyak MA, Moore KA et al (1999) Effects of exercise training on older adults with major depression. Arch Intern Med 159:2349–2356
23. Babyak M, Blumenthal JA, Herman S et al (2000) Exercise treatment for major depression: maintenance of therapeutic benefit at 10 months. Psychosom Med 62:633–638
24. Harari YN (2018) Homo deus. Beck, München
25. Huxley A (2015) Brave new world. Chatto & Windus, London, 1932. German edition: Schöne neue Welt. Fischer, Frankfurt a. M
26. Topol E (2019) Deep Medicine. Basic Books, New York

4

Man: An Underdeveloped Computer?

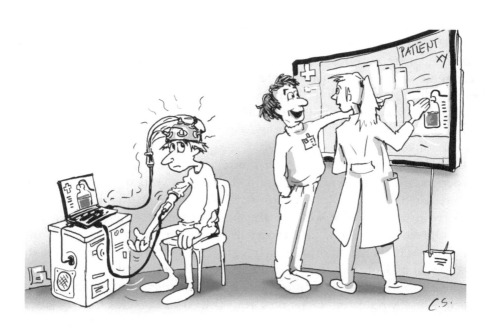

Abstract "Big Data" is the latest big promise of salvation in psychiatry. Here we are promised to be able to diagnose mental illnesses earlier and better and then also to treat them more successfully, if only we have collected enough data about the individual and thus "explained" him. The human being, reduced to his brain, is understood here as a biomachine that can be simulated by an artificial intelligence and whose behaviour can then consequently also be predicted exactly. According to this understanding, the brain is a computer, albeit a less powerful one. However, we are still far away from the realization of such an utopia, and how a therapy can be derived from the insights gained is currently completely in the dark.

Every day we read and hear in the daily press, but also in the medical press, about the promises of "big data", "precision medicine" and "machine learning" for medicine. The first thing one usually reads is that mental illness represents an enormous proportion of the global burden of disease, which is increasing rapidly. I detailed this in Chap. 2. "Estimates put the economic cost [of mental illness] at $2.5 trillion in 2010, and it is expected to double by 2030" [1]. Immediately following this, reference is then made to the seemingly endless possibilities of digitalization in medicine. "Big Data," the analysis and aggregation of ever-increasing amounts of data of every kind collected on every individual, is hailed as the solution to all problems in psychiatry. Not only early detection of mental disorders, but also therapy is supposed to be fundamentally improved as a result. The promises sound heavenly: "The emerging field of 'predictive analytics in mental health' has recently generated tremendous interest with the bold promise to revolutionize clinical practice in psychiatry paralleling similar developments in personalized and precision medicine" [2]. What does this mean? What should this revolution in psychiatry look like?

Parallels are readily drawn with cancer medicine (oncology), which has experienced an enormous upswing in the last ten years due to advances in molecular biology and information technology. Scientists and the lay press alike paint a vision of a world in which no one will ever die of cancer again [3]. Oncologists are now increasingly decoding not only the patient's entire genome, but also that of the tumor, in order to derive a therapy tailored to the individual patient. In addition to the data resulting from the analysis of the genetic material, data are also obtained from all conceivable other sources, such as bodily fluids and excretions, heart (ECG) and brain (EEG) signals, as well as from imaging procedures such as computer tomography (CT) or magnetic resonance imaging (MRI). This "big data" is then analysed using modern machine analysis methods, which are often referred to as "machine learning" or "deep learning". In oncology, significant successes have already been achieved in this way in recent years in the fight against some types of cancer [3]. Now the euphoric hope of being able to detect diseases earlier and treat them better in the future—by combining large amounts of data and their machine analysis—has also reached psychiatry.

The term "digital phenotyping" describes one aspect of this approach. Here, the digital data generated by the use of mainly the smartphone, but also other digital sensors (for example, the motion sensors in today's widely used sports watches), are used to draw conclusions about emotions, mental performance and the behavior of its user. In a paper published in 2015, a typical application of the technology is described as follows: "For a bipolar patient [bipolar disorder = manic-depressive illness; author's note] whose mania [a state of usually elevated mood, heightened drive, and greatly increased activity] manifests itself in rapid, uninterruptible fluency or hypergraphia ["writing a lot"], his illness could be characterized by the frequency, duration, and content of social media participation. Through these multiple applications, digital phenotypes can help ensure that early signs of disease do not go unnoticed and allow the health care system to develop more rapid, targeted, and expedited interventions" [4]. Again, this was pioneered by the former director of the US National Institute of Mental Health, Tom Insel, mentioned in the previous chapter. He moved first to Google in 2015, and later to the Californian startup Mindstrong. On its website, the company promises, "Digital phenotyping is at the core of our measurement approach. Digital phenotyping is simply an assessment based on smartphone usage. As smartphones have become ubiquitous, their increasing use provides an unprecedented opportunity to passively, objectively, and continuously measure mood, perception, and behavior." In an article for a prestigious journal, Insel wrote, "Even though smartphone technology promises to transform many aspects of health care, no area of medicine is likely to be changed more by this technology than psychiatry. Digital phenotyping is the term now used for describing this new approach to measuring behavior from smartphone sensors, keyboard interaction, and various features of voice and speech" [5]. Further, he wrote, "Over the past 4 decades, behavioral expertise, once the strength of psychiatry, has diminished in importance as psychiatric research focused on pharmacology, genomics, and neuroscience, and much of psychiatric practice has become a series of brief clinical interactions focused on medication management. In research settings, assigning a diagnosis from the Diagnostic and Statistical Manual of Mental Disorders, has become a surrogate for behavioral observation. In practice, few clinicians measure emotion, cognition, or behavior with any standard, validated tools" [5]. Insel thus poses nothing less than the hypothesis that the detailed description of psychological experience, as it has been carried out in Germany in particular at the highest scientific level—this is also widely acknowledged internationally, even in the USA—is now to be replaced by the analysis of digital signals that we leave behind with our smartphones, because this allows a more "objective" diagnosis.

It is hoped that the pictures we post on Facebook or Instagram can be used to infer our state of mind. Initial studies have already been published, according to which the diagnoses "depression" or "post-traumatic stress disorder" [abbreviation PTSD, a mental illness caused by psychological trauma] could be made in a high percentage by an algorithm on the basis of Instagram photos or Twitter posts, in some cases long before a clinical diagnosis was made. For example, American researchers have used "machine learning" to develop an algorithm that should be able to determine with high accuracy whether users have depression based on photos posted on Instagram [6]. The diagnostic accuracy is said to be higher than that of general practitioners (although here the diagnostic accuracy was assessed in a different patient population). Photos of depressed individuals tended to be bluer, darker, and grayer. Posts from these individuals received significantly fewer "likes," but they were commented on more frequently than posts from individuals who were not classified as depressed. Interestingly, depressed individuals also posted more frequently than non-depressed individuals. Finally, they also posted photos with faces more frequently, but the number of faces depicted in the photos was lower than in healthy individuals. According to the authors, the algorithm also identified a depressed person more reliably than a general practitioner (again, collected in a different group of people) when only the data posted before diagnosis was considered [6]. These authors also report similar results for short messages posted via the messaging service Twitter [7]. A learning computer program that analyzed 280,000 tweets from 105 depressed and 99 healthy individuals for affect, linguistic style, and context was able to successfully discriminate patients from healthy individuals, and again did so even when the analysis considered only tweets posted prior to diagnosis. Once again, diagnostic accuracy was higher than that of general practitioners, although again this was compared to published data from a different patient population. Finally, using their algorithm, the authors analyzed 244,000 tweets from 174 patients with post-traumatic stress disorder. According to this analysis, evidence of PTSD was found virtually immediately after a trauma, even if the clinical diagnosis had not been made until months later. The authors concluded, "These methods suggest a data-driven, predictive approach to early screening and detection of mental illness." [7]. Currently, all of these machine algorithms have yet to learn on patient populations where the psychiatric diagnosis was previously made by human experts. If a computer is to make diagnoses entirely without such "biases," i.e., true screening on a previously unremarkable group of people, whole new questions arise that do not seem to have been thought through to the end.

However, "Big Data" in psychiatry goes far beyond digital phenotyping. Machines should very soon be able to analyse speech in order to make diagnoses, e.g. of depression or developing dementia. Even the type of music we listen to should allow conclusions to be drawn about our emotional state. But of course, not only our digital data, but also a variety of biological data—genes, hormone levels, everything that can be "measured"—will be included in the analysis. Researchers at the Department of Psychiatry and Psychotherapy at Ludwig Maximilians University in Munich are playing a leading international role. For several years, they have been investigating whether machine learning can be used to determine from anatomical data obtained by magnetic resonance imaging (MRI) whether a subject who is clinically at high risk of developing schizophrenia will actually become ill [8]. The algorithm developed by the researchers on a group of 73 subjects at high risk of developing schizophrenia, i.e. based on brain structure, predicted the risk of developing schizophrenia within the next four years with 80% accuracy. Since 45% of the individuals studied actually developed schizophrenia during the observation period, this result represents a significant gain in diagnostic confidence. However, it should also be noted that the machine predicted transition to schizophrenia in 14% of subjects, but this did not then occur [8]. The hope of this approach, which is promoted as "personalized" or "predictive" medicine—similar to the medicine of physical diseases—is to eventually reduce diagnostic or predictive uncertainty more and more through a whole battery of different biomarkers. The vision that inspires this research is to be able to "discover" mental illnesses so early that they no longer occur at all, because it is possible to intervene at an early stage. The aim is to avoid serious illnesses altogether. However, this concept, which at first seems so simple and promising, raises questions that fundamentally concern human beings in their self-understanding and the structure of future human societies.

In the science fiction film "Minority Report" by Steven Spielberg (2002) is depicted how such a future could look like: The "Precrime" (a nice linguistic analogy to "prediction") division of the Washington Police Department uses "precognition" to prevent murders. The three "precogs," Agatha, Arthur, and Dashiell, have psychic abilities that enable them to predict murders of the future. The police take the potential "perpetrators" (which they are not yet and never will be) into "custody" and place them in a state of permanent unconsciousness. Minority Report is set in 2054, but scientists from China are already showing how close we are to such a vision of the future. Back in 2016, artificial intelligence researchers from Shanghai University presented a study showing that their algorithm can tell with 90% certainty whether someone is a "criminal" from a photo of their face [9]. Although realistic scenarios that could be derived from such research are still far off, comparable studies from other fields suggest that issues of great social consequence are emerging. One example is the recent publication by British scientists according to which their machine learning approach could determine with over 90% certainty from the determination of the activity of genes from the blood [a so-called "gene expression profile"] whether a subject had been sleep deprived the night before [10]. The development of non-invasive [i.e. without injury to tissue, such as occurs through blood sampling], non-blood-based biomarkers will only be a matter of time in order to be able to easily determine whether a person is sufficiently fit to perform their job or participate in road traffic at a given time.

Recently, there has also been discussion about apps that can predict the life expectancy of an individual. Actuaries have been making such calculations for a long time, for example when it comes to calculating whether a person should still be sold life insurance at a certain age in the presence of certain illnesses, and if so, at what price. Today, companies developing such apps promise to make highly customized predictions for individual users by applying Big Data and AI. Primitive data used by such an app (and also by actuaries) includes gender, age, weight, height and ethnicity. In addition, there is occupation, socioeconomic status, and family history regarding certain medical conditions ("Did your parents suffer from high blood pressure or Alzheimer's disease?"). Finally, such an app could track athletic activity and dietary habits. With the proliferation of activity trackers and smartwatches, data from such sensors is now being added, i.e. activity level, heart rate or blood pressure. The sky's the limit in terms of expanding this personal data set. In addition to a full genetic profile that would be made available to the app, any number of laboratory values could be determined in the blood, and when microscopic sensors eventually circle through our bloodstream (this is also already being worked on), this data will be wirelessly and permanently transmitted to the app for continuous monitoring. Proponents of such predictive approaches argue that users could be motivated to adopt healthier lifestyles. Insurers could make personalized offers tailored to the individual's risk. And governments could direct their limited resources where they are needed. But there are risks, too: We will see later that even the (sometimes supposed!) *knowledge of* personal (genetic) disease risk can lead to a change in bodily functions. Knowledge of a low life expectancy could lead to anxiety and depression in some people, and worry could lower life expectancy even more than the physiological data suggest. A scenario in which insurers require clients to submit extensive personal health data before issuing an insurance policy is absolutely realistic. Already, no one gets life insurance unless they have undergone a medical examination and provided detailed information about pre-existing conditions. Above a certain risk score, insurers could refuse insurance altogether, even if the applicant is perfectly healthy and free of pre-existing conditions at the time of application. And governments could also discriminate against individuals or groups of people based on their risk profile, for example by excluding them from certain professions or taxing them differently (more heavily) according to their potential future costs to society. The protection of such highly sensitive data would also be extremely critical, because what the American Internet corporations already know about us today is child's play compared to the explosive power of the data that will be available about every individual in the future. As useful as Big Data approaches can be in the future, if they are used carefully, they all start from a very basic premise: Humans are determined by their genes and biology, and if I have their data as an image of this genetic and biological profile, I know their future.

In "Minority Report", it is crimes that are prevented before they are committed. However, the vision of the future of "Big Data Psychiatry" goes far beyond this, and it opens up many questions: Will it still be doctors who make diagnoses in the future? Or will this be done by the new supercomputers, which in the future will perhaps no longer be located at Google, Amazon or Apple, but at a supreme national health authority? And when the machine has found evidence from all my data that I am at high risk of developing depression, who will be informed? A national health care system? A mental health superintendent? Will I then be contacted by them to seek treatment?

Will I be subject to restrictions if I do not agree to provide my data to the "super predictive computer"? Will I still be able to buy health insurance if I don't agree to do so? At present, such scenarios seem far-fetched, but as the predictive reliability of our diagnostic systems increases, that may quickly change. Mental illnesses represent extremely expensive conditions not only for the healthcare system but also for society as a whole. It is quite possible to envisage societal systems in which the pressure on the individual to undergo preventive treatment in order to avoid costs will be considerable. Will the individual be able to resist this pressure if only predictive certainty is high enough?

Such considerations may seem absurd at present. Any patient, even those with very serious illnesses, can currently withdraw from treatment in any Western country if they do not want it. A person suffering from schizophrenia in Germany, for example, can only be treated against his will if he is a vital danger to himself or others. The hurdles for such compulsory treatment are rightly very high, and as soon as the conditions for such treatment no longer exist, it must be terminated. For example, a patient who a few days ago wanted to take his own life in a delusional misjudgment of his situation can be treated against his will, for example with medication. But as soon as he credibly distances himself from the delusion and suicidal tendencies, he can withdraw from further treatment, even if the risk of a rapid return of the symptoms that led to the suicide attempt is extremely high. In such cases, at least in Western societies, individual freedom, including the freedom to harm oneself, still takes precedence over the community's interest in, for example, minimizing burdens and costs on the health care system. But what will happen when computer algorithms are perfected and predict or pretend to predict a probability of illness that borders on certainty? Biomarkers for suicidal behavior are also being worked on, and again it is expected that in the not too distant future scientists will present profiles of biomarkers that will be used by a computer to calculate probabilities of suicidal behavior through machine learning [11]. If a recent suicide attempt is already enough for me to be treated against my will in a locked psychiatric ward, will it be enough in the future for a computer to certify that I have a 95% risk of suicidal behavior in the next four weeks? Or will I be monitored by the health system (ultimately, again, a computer) on the basis of my digital data traces in order to be able to intervene quickly if necessary?

It is likely that the 80% probability with which the algorithm developed by the Munich scientists is able to predict a person with a high risk of developing schizophrenia will not be sufficient for us to derive more than recommendations for further behaviour and possible further therapy. At what level of certainty do these recommendations become binding? 90%? 95%? Even with such a high degree of certainty, there will be some subjects for whom the machine predicts a transition to schizophrenia, but this then does not occur. In the Munich study, the computer predicted the transition to schizophrenia in 14% of the subjects, which then did not occur. This is certainly a value which does not justify binding demands on the behaviour of the test persons (one should not speak of patients here, because they are not yet ill) or even a therapy. The long observation period of four years must also be taken into account here. The longer the period for which a probability statement is made, the more certain the statements should be, because they may have a considerable influence on the life of the test person. An absolutely certain, binding statement about the occurrence of a certain event, be it the development of schizophrenia or imminent suicide, would only be possible if it could be predicted with 100% certainty. But this would mean that man is an absolutely deterministic biomachine whose future is determined solely by the interaction of his genes and biomolecules—and then, in the final analysis, by his atoms. I will return to the critique of this kind of radical determinism later.

The protagonists of personalised or predictive medicine like to argue that early detection of a disease risk enables early intervention and thus also prevents the development of more severe disease courses. Again, the parallel with cancer medicine is obvious. It is quite obvious that a tumour can be better treated if it is detected at an early stage, before it has spread to neighbouring tissues or even developed metastases. It may even make sense to remove a tissue as a precaution before even an early stage of cancer has developed if there is a very high risk of disease. A very well-known example is that of the American actress Angelina Jolie, who had both breasts removed prophylactically because she is a carrier of a mutation (in the tumor suppressor gene BRCA1) and has a family history of breast cancer. Her risk of developing breast cancer herself was estimated at more than 80%. I will return to this in more detail later, in Chap. 7. But is this situation transferable to psychiatry? To date, we do not know how mental illnesses develop. Ideas that it is a matter of simple biochemical "defects" that could be corrected by a drug have proved far too simplistic. After the discovery of today's antidepressants and antipsychotics in the late 1950s, efforts were made in the following years to understand their molecular mechanisms of action. It was quickly discovered that the antidepressants with which we still treat our patients today increase the concentrations of the neurotransmitters noradrenalin and/or serotonin in the brain. This led to the so-called "catecholamine hypothesis of depression". On the other hand, antipsychotics were found to block the receptors for the neurotransmitter dopamine, from which the "dopamine hypothesis of schizophrenia" was developed. From the molecular mechanisms of action of the—accidentally discovered (!)—psychotropic drugs, hypotheses were developed about the biological causes of mental illness. To date, however, there is no evidence that depression is really caused by a serotonin or norepinephrine deficiency, and the excess of dopamine suspected in schizophrenia is presumably a biological mechanism that is characteristic not only of these disorders and is determined to a large extent by environmental influences such as childhood trauma [12]. It is still completely unclear how the respective complex diseases develop from individual dysfunctions of nerve cells, which have certainly been demonstrated. It is equally unclear how most mental illnesses are cured. Antidepressants and antipsychotics are effective for depression and schizophrenia, and in many cases they are undoubtedly a blessing. However, they do not cure these disorders, and in many cases their effectiveness is also inadequate (as I pointed out above). Thus, while antipsychotics today enable many people with schizophrenia to live again in the community by relieving them of delusions and hallucinations, they are now excluded from employment in the primary labor market—an indicator of social capacity—to an even greater extent than 50 years ago. But we know even less about the treatment that really prevents the onset of a mental illness in a person at risk of developing it. We know quite well what measures we can take to reduce the risk of mental illness in general. However, it has not yet been possible to prove that the precautionary administration of antipsychotics to so-called "high-risk patients" reduces their risk of falling ill. On the other hand, such a "therapy"—which is actually not a therapy, because a disease has not yet occurred—accepts considerable side effects. A truly meaningful predictive diagnosis therefore requires not only a clear understanding of the mechanisms of disease development, but above all a clearly effective therapy. In general, it seems even more absurd to treat people with an increased risk of developing depression with an antidepressant. This could then go so far as to "treat" anyone with such a substance who is caring for a terminally ill relative, because such a situation undoubtedly carries an increased risk of depression. This would then be a further step towards a "cosmetic psychopharmacology", as propagated by the American psychiatrist Peter Kramer in his world bestseller "Listening to Prozac" [13].

The implications of "big data" medicine are even more far-reaching than in somatic medicine when it comes to defining "normality". The extent to which psychiatric diagnoses have changed, even in just a few decades, has been outlined by the influential American psychiatrist Allen Frances in his book "Normal", which is well worth reading [14]. Frances chaired the committee that wrote the fourth version of the American Diagnostic and Statistical Manual of Mental Disorders (DSM-IV), which appeared in 1994. He criticizes the increasing pathologization of the normal with each version of the DSM and the inflationary expansion of psychiatric diagnoses, as culminated for the time being in DSM-5, published in 2013. Frances states that the reformulation of diagnostic criteria in DSM-IV in the years following its publication led to an extreme increase in the diagnoses of "autism", "attention deficit hyperactivity disorder" (ADHD) and "bipolar disorder". With the introduction of DSM-5, more disorders had been "invented" that pathologized behaviors previously thought to be normal. These include "binge-eating disorder", "ADHD in adulthood", "mild neurocognitive deficit" and "behavioural addictions". Each new diagnosis, he said, leads to the need for new treatment, not the least of which is psychotropic drugs. Interestingly, new drugs have been approved for some of these "new" disorders (for example, lisdexamfetamine for binge-eating disorder or atomoxetine for adult ADHD), giving them a virtual monopoly on the treatment of the disorder. A particularly dramatic example of a dangerous expansion of diagnosis is the "invention" of bipolar disorder (formerly manic-depressive illness) in children, which led to children as young as two or three being treated with antipsychotics or lithium in the USA. In many cases, this already set the course for a lifelong patient "career". Severe psychiatric illnesses, such as schizophrenia, mania or severe psychotic depression, are undoubtedly illnesses that have been and continue to be regarded as pathological deviations from "normal" in every age and culture. However, recent decades have led to such an inflationary use of psychiatric diagnoses that one can no longer doubt a significant cultural and social influence on the concept of "mental illness." How else can it be explained that the incidence of bipolar disorder in childhood and adolescence increased 40-fold [15] and that of autism 20-fold [16] in less than two decades? But if much of the diagnostic process in psychiatry remains highly subjective, ultimately based on the consensus of a few experts who every few years redefine the criteria that constitute a particular disorder, then who defines the boundary between "healthy" and "sick"? Psychological experience, as a fundamentally *subjective* experience, cannot in principle be objectified, which is why all attempts to identify clear "biomarkers" for any mental illness have so far failed. If a computer now identifies indications from a person's digital (or other) data that a mental illness could develop in the future: Who draws the line between "healthy" and "sick"? The machine? On the basis of probability statements? At what probability is intervention mandatory? 90%? 99%? And if we believe—as some actually do, for whom man is a deterministic biomachine—that the disease is 100% certain to occur, what then? Do we treat it "prophylactically" in the sense of "preventive" medicine? Do we have a right to warn a (future) "patient" even if we have a therapy available that is reasonably certain to prevent the onset of the disease (which is not the case at the moment)? At what point is "depression" in need of treatment if it is diagnosed by a machine? After all, even the machine has to make a diagnosis based on criteria—who sets those? Even in the diagnosis of physical illnesses, where the situation seems to be clearer because it can be measured "objectively" (e.g. laboratory values), these questions arise. For example, in a recent article worth reading, scholars at the prestigious American universities of Harvard and Stanford asked the question, "Who is normal in the era of precision medicine and Big Data?" [17].

The protagonists of "precision medicine" gave the answer to these questions several years ago (with the concept of the so-called "Research Domain Criteria", RDoC). The pioneer here was also Tom Insel, still during his time at the American NIMH. He propagated that the American diagnostic system (the DSM, see above), which was based purely on expert consensus, had to be replaced by a biologically defined diagnostic system. The DSM was purely oriented towards reliability, i.e. verifiability and communicability. Reliability refers to the reliability of a measurement. A test is reliable if different examiners arrive at the same result. The goal of the DSM was that clinicians in different cultures and contexts should arrive at the same diagnosis if they had the same patient in front of them. In this respect, the DSM—as well as the parallel diagnostic system of the WHO ICD 10—was and is very successful. Insel accused this system of sacrificing validity for this purpose. Validity is a measure of the accuracy with which the trait is actually measured that is intended to be measured. Insel wrote on his blog in May 2013 when the latest edition of the DSM (DSM-5) was released: "The strength of each of the editions of DSM has been "reliability"—each edition has ensured that clinicians use the same terms in the same ways. The weakness is its lack of validity. Unlike our definitions of ischemic heart disease, lymphoma, or AIDS, the DSM diagnoses are based on a consensus about clusters of clinical symptoms, not any objective laboratory measure. In the rest of medicine, this would be equivalent to creating diagnostic systems based on the nature of chest pain or the quality of fever. Indeed, symptom-based diagnosis, once common in other areas of medicine, has been largely replaced in the past half century as we have understood that symptoms alone rarely indicate the best choice of treatment." He continued, "Patients with mental disorders deserve better. The NIMH has launched the Research Domain Criteria (RDoC) project to transform diagnosis by incorporating genetics, imaging, cognitive science, and other levels of information to lay the foundation for a new classification system" [18].

The vision of this concept is therefore to make diagnoses in the future on the basis of biomarker profiles. The concept suggests that in the future—perhaps somewhat exaggeratedly formulated—we will no longer treat the suffering person, but the disturbed brain function. Do we then "treat" the biomarker profile? Or the person who may not (yet) be suffering at all? Will there be thresholds, as is common with lab values, outside of which we should advise treatment? How do we even treat when we still have no clear idea of how mental illness develops? In fact, large parts of academic psychiatry are convinced that we only need to characterize the "defect" in the brains of our patients (and then consequently also in still healthy people) more precisely in order to be able to treat them better in the future.

"Big Data" approaches such as digital phenotyping unfortunately completely ignore the fact that in a hierarchically organized system, more complex structures ("psyche") cannot necessarily be explained by the laws of subordinate organizational levels (genes, neurons). In its efforts to become a serious discipline based on the natural sciences, psychiatry has moved ever closer to the prevailing thinking in medicine. After the failure of a radical biological approach, according to which healthy as well as ill mental experience is determined by biological processes and thus ultimately by the programme of our genes, behaviour is now explained in a "biopsychosocial model" by the more or less complex interactions between genes and environment. The relatively new science of epigenetics in psychiatry in particular is now attempting to explain how environmental influences affect the expression of genes and thus in turn our neurobiology by studying "gene-environment interactions". Even according to this conception, however, humans are determined by these interactions, since they do not occur as their active shapers. According to this conception of the world, mental processes are only epiphenomena of the gene-environment interaction, whereby the brain is conceived here merely as a mediating instance. An epiphenomenon is a phenomenon that is causally produced (here, for example, by the activity of nerve cells), but does not itself exert a causal effect. Concepts such as that of "emergence", according to which in a system developing to ever higher degrees of complexity the properties of higher levels of organisation cannot be explained by the laws of the systems arranged hierarchically below them, have lost considerable importance after the peak of their popularity in the 1980s and 90s (in the context of the so-called "New Age" movement). The American philosopher and social scientist Donald Campbell coined the principle of "downward causation", according to which in hierarchical systems a complex structure can have an effect on its components [19]. According to this principle, humans influence their biology by changing themselves and their social structures.

An excellent example of downward causality is placebo and nocebo effects. These effects summarize all the effects of the context that influence the effects of a drug. It is never the biological effect of a drug alone that determines its effectiveness, but the totality of numerous environmental factors. Among these, the patient's expectation of the effect of a drug plays a particularly significant role. If the patient (or test person) expects negative effects from the preparation he or she is taking, and if these then actually occur as side effects (although he or she has only received a placebo preparation), this is known as the nocebo effect. So while the placebo effect describes the apparent positive effects of a drug, the nocebo effect encompasses the apparent negative effects. Interestingly, the placebo effect in clinical trials of psychotropic drugs has increased over the decades since their introduction. For example, scientists from the Technical University of Munich have shown that in the testing of antipsychotics (drugs for psychosis, especially schizophrenia), the effect of the real drug (the so-called "verum", i.e. the "true" substance) has remained stable over the years, but the effectiveness of the placebo has increased more and more, so that in the last ten to twenty years it has become increasingly difficult to show the superiority of an antipsychotic over placebo [20]. To date, it is unclear what the environmental factors are that cause patients to respond to a drug that does not contain a biologically active agent. However, it appears that the context in which we treat has changed (positively) to such an extent that the treatment itself, without administration of a verum, improves the treatment outcome. Equally remarkable is that even the placebo effect is subject to biological and even genetic influences. Genetic variants are now known to influence the magnitude of the placebo effect in a defined individual [21]. At the same time, it is possible to specifically block the placebo effect pharmacologically: for example, if a subject expects to be given a painkiller, the analgesic effect, which can also be achieved by a placebo, can be reduced by the administration of an opiate antagonist (i.e., a drug that blocks the effects of potent painkillers). This suggests that the expectation of receiving an analgesic addresses the same biological mechanism as the analgesic itself [22]. However, how the "psyche" or "consciousness" interacts with the brain here is as unclear as the mechanisms that lead to changes in our emotions, mood, or perception via modulation of neurotransmitters that nerve cells use to communicate with each other, such as serotonin.

Finally, in the discussion about how mental illnesses should be diagnosed and then treated, it is often forgotten that emotions such as depression, fear or despair have their evolutionary meaning. Western industrial societies in particular tend to regard these as undesirable and to want to eliminate them at all costs. According to the DSM-5, even prolonged grief after the loss of a partner is now considered an illness. The tendency to want to turn off unpleasant feelings is one reason why the use (or perhaps better consumption?) of antidepressants has increased dramatically in the last twenty years and continues to increase every year, as we have seen above. Evolutionarily, however, these feelings have the purpose of changing our situation, they signal that our circumstances are perceived as needing improvement. The example of the rat, which has become apathetic towards the well-being of its fellow species, signals that trying to turn off unwanted feelings with a drug is not necessarily the best solution.

"Big Data", "Deep Learning" or "digital phenotyping" will certainly provide us with many new insights into the functioning of our brain and probably also into the development of mental disorders. A sole focus of academic psychiatry on these explanatory approaches reduces the human being to a biomachine that is determined by its genes, molecules and then ultimately even by its digital signals. This gives people a self-image that deprives them of the freedom to shape their own future. This situation causes many people at least as much discomfort as the developments that have led to the epidemic increase in the prescription of antidepressants themselves.

References

1. Conway M, O'Connor D (2016) Social media, big data, and mental health: current advances and ethical implications. Curr Opin Psychol 9:77–82
2. Hahn T, Nierenberg AA, Whitfield-Gabrieli S (2017) Predictive analytics in mental health: applications, guidelines, challenges and perspectives. Mol Psychiatry 22:37–43
3. Schulz T (2018) Zukunftsmedizin. Deutsche Verlagsanstalt, München
4. Jain SH, Powers BW, Hawkins JB, Brownstein JS (2015) The digital phenotype. Nat Biotechnol 33:462–463
5. Insel TR (2017) Digital phenotyping: technology for a new science of behavior. JAMA 318:1215–1216
6. Reece AG, Danforth CM (2017) Instagram photos reveal predictive markers of depression. EPJ Data Sci 6:15
7. Reece AG, Reagan AJ, Lix KLM et al (2017) Forecasting the onset and course of mental illness with Twitter data. Sci Rep 7:13006
8. Koutsouleris N, Riecher-Rössler A, Meisenzahl EM et al (2015) Detecting the psychosis prodrome across high-risk populations using neuroanatomical biomarkers. Schizophr Bull 41:471–482
9. Süddeutsche Zeitung. Neue Software soll Kriminelle an ihren Gesichtszügen erkennen. November 27th 2016. https://www.sueddeutsche.de/panorama/verbrechen-im-namen-der-nase-1.3268675. Accessed on May 8th 2020
10. Laing EE, Möller-Levet CS, Dijk DJ, Archer SN (2019) Identifying and validating blood mRNA biomarkers for acute and chronic insufficient sleep in humans: a machine learning approach. Sleep 42:zsy186
11. Niculescu AB, Le-Niculescu H, Levey DF et al (2017) Precision medicine for suicidality: from universality to subtypes and personalization. Mol Psychiatry 22:1250–1273
12. Egerton A, Valmaggia LR, Howes OD et al (2016) Adversity in childhood linked to elevated striatal dopamine function in adulthood. Schizophr Res 176:171–176
13. Kramer PD (1997) Listening to prozac: a psychiatrist explores antidepressant drugs and the remaking of the self. Penguin Books, revised 1997
14. Frances A (2013) Saving normal. An insider's revolt against out-of-control psychiatric daignosis, DSM-5, big pharma, and the medicalization of ordinary life. HarperCollins Publishers, New York
15. Moreno C, Laje G, Blanco C et al (2007) National trends in the outpatient diagnosis and treatment in youth. Arch Gen Psychiatry 64:1032–1039
16. Centers for Disease Control and Prevention (CDC). CDC estimates 1 in 88 children in the United States has been identified as having an autism spectrum disorder. (https://www.cdc.gov/media/releases/2012/p0329_autism_disorder.html. Accessed on May 8, 2020

17. Manrai AK, Patel CJ, Ioannidis JPA (2018) In the era of precision medicine and big data, who is normal? JAMA 319:1981–1982
18. Insel T (2013) Post by Former NIMH Director Thomas Insel: Transforming Diagnosis. April 29th 2013. https://www.nimh.nih.gov/about/directors/thomas-insel/blog/2013/transforming-diagnosis.shtml. Accessed on May 8th 2020
19. Campbell DT (1974) Downward causation in hierarchically organised biological systems. In: Ayala F, Ayala FJ, Ayala FJ, Dobzhansky T (Hrsg) Studies in the philosophy of biology: reduction and related problems. Macmillan, London/Basingstoke, S 179–186
20. Leucht S, Leucht C, Huhn M et al (2017) Sixty years of placebo-controlled antipsychotic drug trials in acute schizophrenia: systematic review, Bayesian meta-analysis, and meta-regression of efficacy predictors. Am J Psychiatry 174:927–942
21. Furmark T, Appel L, Henningsson S et al (2008) A link between serotonin-related gene polymorphisms, amygdala activity, and placebo-induced relief from social anxiety. J Neurosci 28:13066–13074
22. Benedetti F, Mayberg HS, Wager TD, Stohler CS, Zubieta JK (2005) Neurobiological mechanisms of the placebo effect. J Neurosci 25:10390–10402

Part II

Why Biology Is Not Destiny

5

Widespread Diseases of the Twenty-First Century

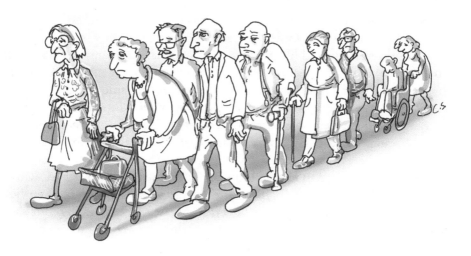

Abstract Dementias and depressions are among the major widespread diseases of the twenty-first century, whose significance is constantly growing in ever ageing populations. The most effective measures to prevent them are not therapeutic but prophylactic. At the same time, these measures also increase physical and psychological well-being and they preserve cognitive performance. New estimates suggest that 30% of all dementias are preventable through lifestyle changes. Protective lifestyle factors include education, avoidance of obesity, physical activity, avoidance of smoking, normalization of blood pressure and blood sugar, maintenance of social relationships, and treatment of depression and hearing loss.

© Springer-Verlag GmbH Germany, part of Springer Nature 2022
G. Gründer, *How Do We Want to Live?*, https://doi.org/10.1007/978-3-662-64225-2_5

The way to better mental and physical health is not to treat health disorders that have already occurred. The simplest and, moreover, most effective means of avoiding disease is to prevent it. In many areas of medicine and public health, this is a truism. For example, the major infectious diseases of human history, to which millions of people fell victim, were not defeated by better treatment options (e.g. drugs such as antibiotics), but by hygienic and pro-phylactic interventions. This also applies to many of today's widespread dis-eases, which we also like to call diseases of civilization. For example, once depression has developed, it can be arduous and protracted to overcome it, and the risk of relapse after a depressive episode is not small. In everyday life, this is even more obvious when it comes to body weight. Anyone who has ever tried not only to reduce an elevated body weight but also to maintain it in the long term knows this. This is even more true in the case of cancer. The com-parison may seem absurd at first glance, but unfortunately it is still far too little known that the individual risk of cancer can also be influenced very significantly by lifestyle factors. Once a cancer has developed, however, con-siderable effort and strain must be endured in order to overcome it.

Here, however, I would like to go one step further. The same behaviors and actions that reduce the risk of health problems occurring also help increase physical and mental health and well-being. It's not the same thing. It is much easier to motivate yourself to behave or change your behaviour if you realise that you can not only prevent some event (the onset of illness) but increase your cur-rent wellbeing. "Well-being" is, of course, hard to measure. However, I will present here the evidence that simple behavioral changes that can be imple-mented by anyone lead to longer, healthier, and probably happier lives. This is not about "self-optimization." The desire for "self-optimization" is often held against people who live a healthier lifestyle, exercise and eat healthy. But these are the first and most important measures to counteract many of the widespread diseases that are rampant today, including such stressful ones that rob the people affected of any quality of life, such as depression. And only those who are healthy and cognitively capable, who can feel joy in life, live consciously and do not have to worry every day about their physical or psychological survival, can take care of solving the great problems of mankind, and only then will there be the freedom to develop an eye for the people around them. I would like to explain this in more detail here using the example of dementia.

For many people, the prospect of developing dementia in old age and thus no longer being able to live independently is a terrifying scenario. But even the risk of falling victim to such a dementia can be significantly reduced by simple behavioural changes. A major review paper entitled "Dementia prevention, intervention and care", which appeared some time ago in one of the most pres-tigious medical journals, described dementia as the "greatest global challenge to health and social systems in the twenty-first century" [1]. Since dementias occur mainly in people over 65 years of age and their incidence (number of new cases in a defined population per unit time) increases with age, the increase in the number of people with a dementia-related illness is due to the increase in life expectancy observed worldwide. Globally, approximately 47 million people had dementia in 2015, and current projections are that this number will triple by 2050. The cost of this was about US$ 818 billion, and this figure will also increase dramatically in line with the increase in prevalence (the number of people with the disease per population, calculated as the ratio of the number of people affected in a population to the number of all people in that population; i.e. incidence is a measure of the number of new cases, prevalence is a measure of the number of people with the disease). However, the greater part—about 85%—of these costs is not caused by the medical treatment of the sick, but by the burden on families and social systems. The burden on family members and care institutions in particular is very considerable, because the care of dementia patients, especially with increasing severity of the disease, requires the presence of a caregiver at all times.

Interestingly, some recent studies show that the incidence of dementia has been declining in many countries in recent years. Although prevalence is increasing in all societies as they grow older, the number of new cases in relation to the respective age group is decreasing in some industrialized countries. For example, figures from the famous Framingham Heart study, which began in 1948 to follow the health of a collective of more than 5000 individuals over the long term (and has since included more than 5000 first-generation descendants of subjects), show that the number of new cases of dementia in a defined age group declined substantially over the decades [2]. Between the late 1970s and the mid-2000s, age-specific dementia incidence decreased by more than 40%, and the median age of onset increased by five years, from 80 to 85 years. In parallel, the incidence of most vascular risk factors for dementia (which they are, follows below), with the exception of obesity and diabetes, decreased. However, these parallel trends were only seen in subjects who had at least a high school diploma. This already suggests the importance of education as a protective factor. Vascular risk factors were treated with medication much more frequently in the 2000s than in the 1970s. Whereas in the latter period only 33% of subjects over 60 years of age were taking a medication to lower blood pressure, 30 years later this figure had risen to 62%. Almost one in two (43%) of those over 60 took a drug to lower their cholesterol in the 2000s. These drugs were not even available in the 1970s. The percentage of smokers had also decreased significantly, from 20% to only 6% [2].

There is thus much evidence to suggest that people over the age of 65 in some industrialized nations are now cognitively healthier and more efficient than cohorts of the same age in previous generations [3]. The most likely cause of this decrease in age-specific incidence of dementia is changes in life-style factors, that is, reductions in risk factors and/or increases in protective factors. Thus, it is estimated [1] that more than one third of all dementias could be avoided if preventive measures were taken. While there are biological, primarily genetic factors whose influence on the risk of dementia—at least at present—cannot be influenced (above all ApoE ε4, see Chap. 7), numerous risk factors are now known that can be modified. Thus, contrary to what was believed 10–20 years ago, dementia is no longer a matter of fate. Systematic modification of certain lifestyle factors could mean that many people no longer experience the decline in their cognitive performance. But even postponing the onset of the disease by only a few years and for only a smaller proportion of the population would represent a significant advance for many individuals, as well as for societies, social systems and economies. What is known about this today? Seven risk factors can be identified that are modifiable, and two others (hearing loss and social isolation) have also recently been identified as possible risk factors.

Education Education is a central theme of this book. Education is the pre-requisite for consciously shaping one's own and ultimately the future of the planet. It is not surprising that education is also an important protective fac-tor against the development of dementia. Since the level of education is rela-tively low across all countries in the world, lack of education is one of the most important risk factors for the development of dementia when viewed from a global perspective. Education increases the so-called "cognitive reserve" [4]. People with high cognitive reserve are able to compensate for structural, neuropathological brain changes associated with dementias (e.g., deposits of Alzheimer-specific proteins in the brain) without showing cognitive or func-tional deficits. This means that a person who has a high level of education may show histopathological changes typical of Alzheimer's disease when their brain is examined without being cognitively or functionally impaired, whereas a person with the same structural brain changes who has a low level of educa-tion may already have dementia syndrome.

Overweight and Obesity (see also Chap. 2) Overweight (BMI 25–30 kg/m^2) and obesity (BMI > 30 kg/m^2) are risk factors for both the development of dementia and depression. However, current predictions of future trends in the number of dementia cases do not take this into account. If the increase in overweight and obesity in middle age (in old age, obesity can no longer be identified as a risk factor), as seen in almost all countries around the world, is included in the calculations, this leads to an increase in the number of dementias of 9% in the USA and as much as 19% in China [5]. For Australia, it has been calculated that there will be 14% more dementia cases in 2050 if the trend of increasing overweight and obesity in middle age is taken into account [6]. On the other hand, if the prevalence of obesity was reduced to 20% and the proportion of normal weight increased to 40% between 2015 and 2025, the number of dementia cases in the 65–69 age group could be reduced by 10% in 2050. This is an optimistic scenario, given that in 2010 33% of male Australians and 30% of female Australians had a BMI above 30 and were therefore considered obese.

Physical Inactivity While there are no controlled, prospective studies (that would be studies in which half of the subjects engage in a certain minimum amount of exercise, the other half would engage in little exercise; after a certain period of time, certainly a few years, all subjects would then be examined for their cognitive performance) that show that physical activity halts the loss of cognitive performance with age, observational studies suggest this. A meta-analysis of 15 studies involving nearly 38,000 healthy people who did not have dementia and were followed for up to 12 years demonstrated an inverse relationship between physical activity levels and risk of cognitive impairment. Subjects with the most pronounced activity had the lowest risk, with about a 40% risk reduction over the group that exercised the least. However, even low to moderate physical activity significantly reduced risk [7]. Another meta-analysis of 16 studies involving nearly 164,000 healthy individuals examined the impact of physical activity on the risk of developing a neurodegenerative disease (dementia in general, Alzheimer's dementia, Parkinson's disease). Subjects with the highest level of physical activity had about 30% lower risk of developing dementia and 45% lower risk of developing Alzheimer's dementia compared to subjects with the lowest level of physical activity [8]. People who are physically active fall less often, their mood is better and they live more independently [1].

Smoking While nicotine may have beneficial short-term effects on concentration and attention, smoking is among the most significant risk factors for the development of cognitive impairment and dementia. The effect is certainly due in large part to the negative effects of smoking on cardiovascular function. However, tobacco smoke also contains neurotoxic substances that additionally increase the risk of cognitive impairment [9].

High Blood Pressure (in Middle Age) High blood pressure in middle age is a significant risk factor for the development of dementia. Along with smoking and diabetes, it is one of the important vascular risk factors.

Diabetes Mellitus The importance of diabetes as a dementia risk factor has been increasing for decades because it is becoming more common with the increase in overweight and obesity. In the Framingham Heart study (see above), 10% of those over 60 suffered from type II diabetes (which is the form that is a consequence of obesity) in the late 1970s, and by the mid-2000s this figure had risen to 17% [2]. Different mechanisms are likely to be responsible for diabetes leading to an increased risk of developing dementia, but the link is thought to be established.

Depression There has long been intense debate about whether depressive episodes are a risk factor for developing dementia or whether they are early signs of a developing dementia syndrome. Depression is associated with a reduction in nerve growth factors (such as Brain Derived Neurotrophic Factor, BDNF) and a reduction in the volume of the hippocampus (a brain structure that holds central memory functions), so a causal link seems likely. To investigate this question, a British-French research group studied more than 10,000 people over a period of nearly 30 years (1985–2015). Of the people included in the study in 1985, 322 developed dementia by 2015. Neither the people who were already suffering from depression in 1985 nor those who developed repeated depressive episodes in the first 20 years of the observation period had an increased risk of dementia. However, those who either had depression in 2003 or had recurrent episodes of the condition in the last 11 years of the observation period had about a 70% higher risk of having dementia in 2015. The authors concluded that depression, or even recurrent depressive episodes, did not increase the risk of dementia; rather, they represented a prodrome of developing dementia. Another explanation could be that both disorders have common causes [10]. Interestingly, it has been shown—also in humans—that treatment with antidepressants from the group of selective serotonin reuptake inhibitors (SSRIs) reduces the deposition of the protein plaques typical of AD (the so-called amyloid) [11, 12]. Since the prescription of antidepressants has approximately doubled in all industrialized nations over the past 20 years, if amyloid deposition indeed plays a causal role in the development of AD, this should lead to a decrease in the number of new cases. However, recent epidemiological work shows that this does not seem to be the case. On the contrary, some studies suggest an association between the use of at least some specific antidepressants and an increased risk of dementia [13, 14]. Thus, many unanswered questions remain to be clarified here.

Social Isolation Similar to depression, social isolation (or simply "loneliness") can be debated as to whether it is a real risk factor or rather precedes a developing dementia as a prodromal symptom. Again, of course, social withdrawal can also be a symptom of depression on the one hand, and a risk factor for developing it on the other. Social isolation also increases the risk of developing numerous physical illnesses such as high blood pressure or coronary heart disease. In any case, the data are similarly clear as in the case of depressive disorders. A meta-analysis of 19 longitudinal cohort studies concluded that a lack of social relationships and loneliness were associated with a higher risk of developing dementia [15]. I will return to this topic in the third part of this book.

Hearing Loss Who would have thought that hearing loss is a risk factor for cognitive decline? Although the presence of hearing loss increases the risk of developing dementia quite significantly, its importance has only been recognized in recent years. However, several studies suggest a link. In the Baltimore Longitudinal Study of Aging, 639 healthy individuals underwent hearing tests between 1990 and 1994. By 2008, i.e. after a mean observation period of 12 years, 58 people had developed dementia, 37 of them Alzheimer's dementia. The risk of developing the disease increased with the degree of hearing loss at the beginning of the observation period, and subjects who suffered from severe hearing loss at the beginning had a fivefold increased risk of developing dementia [16]. However, comparable to the risk factors depression and loneliness, it is also unclear in the case of hearing loss whether it is a true risk factor or a very early symptom of the onset of dementia. Only in the first case would treatment of the hearing loss, e.g. by fitting a hearing aid, reduce the risk. However, studies investigating the effects of hearing loss treatment on dementia risk are still pending.

Interestingly, people with hearing loss who seek treatment for it are also particularly likely to suffer from loneliness [17]. Whether there is an (obvious) causal relationship here is unclear, but two risk factors come together here, each of which increases the risk of dementia.

Of course, other risk factors cannot be strictly separated. They are also linked by other factors that the Lancet Commission has not taken into account at all. These include, in particular, diet. In the next chapter I have collected numerous studies which indicate quite clearly that a diet which is lower in meat, plant-based or Mediterranean, can reduce the risk of developing dementia. Such a diet also reduces the risk of high blood pressure, obesity and diabetes mellitus. The protective effects of individual measures, such as physical activity or a healthy diet, therefore reduce the effects of various risk factors.

These two lifestyle factors in particular, i.e. exercise and diet, not only reduce the risk of developing dementia; they are also extremely important for our physical and mental well-being in general. Then there are meditation and other mindfulness techniques. In the last few years in particular, numerous studies have appeared to prove this. The most important findings are discussed in the following chapter.

References

1. Livingston G, Sommerlad A, Orgeta V et al (2017) Dementia prevention, intervention, and care. Lancet 390:2673–2734
2. Satizabal CL, Beiser AS, Chouraki V et al (2016) Incidence of dementia over three decades in the framingham heart study. N Engl J Med 374:523–532
3. Wu YT, Beiser AS, Breteler MMB et al (2017) The changing prevalence and incidence of dementia over time – current evidence. Nat Rev Neurol 13:327–339
4. Stern Y (2012) Cognitive reserve in ageing and Alzheimer's disease. Lancet Neurol 11:1006–1012
5. Loef M, Walach H (2013) Midlife obesity and dementia: meta-analysis and adjusted forecast of dementia prevalence in the United States and China. Obesity (Silver Spring) 21:E51–E55
6. Nepal B, Brown LJ, Anstey KJ (2014) Rising midlife obesity will worsen future prevalence of dementia. PLoS One 9:e99305
7. Sofi F, Valecchi D, Bacci D et al (2011) Physical activity and risk of cognitive decline: a meta-analysis of prospective studies. J Intern Med 269:107–117
8. Hamer M, Chida Y (2009) Physical activity and risk of neurodegenerative disease: a systematic review of prospective evidence. Psychol Med 39:3–11
9. Swan GE, Lessov-Schlaggar CN (2007) The effects of tobacco smoke and nicotine on cognition and the brain. Neuropsychol Rev 17:259–273
10. Singh-Manoux A, Dugravot A, Fournier A et al (2017) Trajectories of depressive symptoms before diagnosis of dementia: a 28-Year follow-up study. JAMA Psychiatry 74:712–718
11. Cirrito JR, Disabato BM, Restivo JL et al (2011) Serotonin signaling is associated with lower amyloid-β levels and plaques in transgenic mice and humans. Proc Natl Acad Sci USA 108:14968–14973
12. Sheline YI, West T, Yarasheski K et al (2014) An antidepressant decreases CSF Aβ production in healthy individuals and in transgenic AD mice. Sci Transl Med:6:236re4
13. Heath L, Gray SL, Boudreau DM et al (2018) Cumulative antidepressant use and risk of dementia in a prospective cohort study. J Am Geriatr Soc 66:1948–1955
14. Wang YC, Tai PA, Poly TN et al (2018) Increased risk of dementia in patients with antidepressants: a meta-analysis of observational studies. Behav Neurol 2018:5315098
15. Kuiper JS, Zuidersma M, Oude Voshaar RC et al (2015) Social relationships and risk of dementia: a systematic review and meta-analysis of longitudinal cohort studies. Ageing Res Rev 22:39–57
16. Lin FR, Metter EJ, O'Brien RJ et al (2011) Hearing loss and incident dementia. Arch Neurol 68:214–220
17. Sung YK, Li L, Blake C, Betz J, Lin FR (2016) Association of hearing loss and loneliness in older adults. J Aging Health 28:979–994

6

Health and Well-Being: What Can Everyone Do?

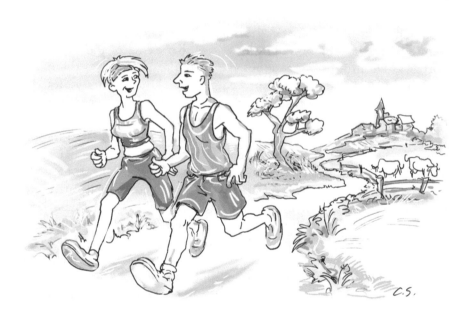

Abstract Nothing has as well proven effects on physical and mental health as physical activity, it doesn't even have to be sport. Exercise not only reduces the risks of cardiovascular disease, strokes and numerous cancers and reduces mortality, it also reduces the risks of dementia and depression and maintains mental performance. The second major lifestyle factor, whose importance not only to our physical health but also to our mental well-being and cognitive performance cannot be overestimated, is diet. Caloric restriction and a plant-based diet low in animal fat and meat have the most significant, empirically proven effects. Mindfulness-based meditation techniques complement interventions for maintaining and enhancing mental health.

Physical Activity

The positive effects of exercise—we don't even necessarily have to talk about sport here—are clearly proven. Even regular light exercise reduces the risks of cardiovascular diseases, strokes and numerous cancers, and mortality decreases overall. Our sedentary lifestyle has depressing effects in every one of these respects. Even in ancient times, doctors as far back as Hippocrates knew about the health benefits of exercise. Plato had written, "A lack of activity impairs the good condition of every man, while exercise and methodical physical training protect and preserve it." This insight was later lost; as late as the mid-twentieth century, the prevailing view was that exercise, and even more so sport, was harmful by wearing out the body prematurely [1]. Hundreds of individual studies have since disproved this view. The sedentary lifestyle that has spread around the world is now considered one of the biggest health risks. In a remarkable analysis, scientists from Harvard University in Boston have calculated how many cases of illness and death can be attributed to our lack of exercise alone [2]. The scientists conclude that 6% of the global burden of disease from coronary heart disease (i.e., narrowing of the coronary arteries due to atherosclerosis) and 7% from type 2 diabetes can be attributed to physical inactivity alone. But even more remarkable—and much less well known—are the figures for the most common cancers: 10% each of the burden of disease from breast cancer and colon cancer—two of the most common types of cancer—can also be explained by lack of exercise alone. Worldwide, 57 million people died in 2008. 9% of those deaths, or 5.3 million, were due to physical inactivity. If physical inactivity were completely eliminated, the global average life expectancy would suddenly increase by 0.68 years [2]. Physical inactivity is a worldwide problem, not only in the highly industrialized Western countries. The Arab states of the eastern Mediterranean region are particularly affected. In countries such as Kuwait, the United Arab Emirates or Saudi Arabia, 17–18% of deaths and around 20% of the two above-mentioned cancers are the result of physical inactivity. In Saudi Arabia, life expectancy would increase by 1.5 years if physical inactivity were eliminated.

The numbers seem comparatively low. Are eight months of life gained worth the effort? Here you have to take into account that the figures represent an average value and apply to the entire world population, i.e. active as well as inactive. If only the inactive population is examined, their gain from taking up physical activity would be significantly greater. It can then amount to up to four years, which is an average of about 5% of the total current lifespan [3].

But what does "lack of exercise" mean in concrete terms? Do we have to exercise excessively in order to benefit from the positive effects on our health? The World Health Organization has published recommendations on this subject [4]. For adults aged 18–64 years, it recommends 150 min of moderate-intensity aerobic activity per week or 75 min of high-intensity aerobic activity, or an appropriate combination of both. "Aerobic activity" is exercise in which the body always works with sufficient oxygen and there is no buildup of what is called "oxygen debt." During this moderate-intensity exercise, fats and carbohydrates are processed, and the cardiovascular system is exercised. For additional positive health effects, the WHO recommends doubling the times mentioned. In addition, exercises to strengthen the large muscle groups are recommended twice a week [4]. These times sound challenging: 150 min of moderate-intensity exercise per week means 30 min of time investment per day, five days a week, if you don't like to really exert yourself for fifteen minutes each on as many days of the week. Are shorter times possibly sufficient to benefit health-wise? This question was posed by a team of Taiwanese researchers, who published their findings in the British Lancet in 2011 [3]. These scientists argue that for Asians in particular, who exercise even less than Americans, a duration of 30 min daily is a significant barrier that leads to such recommendations being disregarded. They therefore studied more than 400,000 people using a questionnaire and divided them into five groups according to their physical activity: inactive, low, moderate, high and very high activity. The health of this huge cohort was then followed for an average of eight years. The results were compelling: even the people in the lowest activity level group, which averaged 92 min per week or 15 min per day, were 14% less likely to die, and their life expectancy was three years longer than the completely inactive group. Each additional quarter of an hour of physical activity per day reduced the probability of death by a further 4% and the probability of death from cancer by 1% [3].

Particularly convincing evidence for the health benefits of physical activity was provided by the Copenhagen City Heart Study. In this study, too, a large sample of the Copenhagen population of almost 20,000 people between the ages of 20 and 98 has been followed over the long term and repeatedly examined and surveyed since 1976. About 10% of this group were classified as joggers. Over the observation period of up to 35 years, 122 of the joggers died, but about 10,000 of the non-joggers died. From these numbers, the researchers calculated a 44% reduced risk of death for the joggers at the same age. The joggers had an increased life expectancy of 6.2 years (men) and 5.6 years (women) [5]. Six years! That's a long time, especially if you can spend it in good health. In the study, the joggers were also significantly less affected by coronary heart disease. However, it is likely that the case numbers in this study were ultimately too small to show a reduction in mortality from cancer. The Copenhagen City Heart Study also provided another important piece of evidence about the right amount of physical activity to benefit from health-wise. Running had the most beneficial effects at low to moderate speeds (about 5 miles per hour, or 8 km per hour) and a frequency of three times per week for a total duration of 60 to 150 min. At very intense running, long durations, or high speeds (7 miles/h = 11.2 km/h), the beneficial effects decreased or were even no longer detectable compared with non-joggers [5, 6].

As indicated in Chap. 3, there are now also numerous studies that show the effectiveness of exercise even in mild to moderate depression, and meta-analyses (these are studies that combine the results of numerous individual studies) also demonstrate the effectiveness of exercise or sport in depressive disorders. Physical activity triggers numerous hormonal and metabolic processes that not only lead to increased metabolic activity and better weight regulation, but also increase psychological well-being. In the brain, messenger substances are released that already acutely lead to a feeling of well-being. In addition, the concentrations of growth factors increase, which stimulate the nerve cells to form new synapses (these are the connection points between nerve cells). This in turn leads to better mental performance and reduces the risks of depression and dementia.

The most significant study that examined the relationship between physical activity and mental health was published in 2018 in the prestigious journal *Lancet Psychiatry* [7]. In this study, more than 1.2 million people in the U.S. were asked about their mental health between 2011 and 2015 with the following question: "Thinking about your mental health, which includes stress, depression, or even emotional problems, how many days in the past 30 days was your mental health not good?" Subjects were also asked about their physical activity in the past month, "In the past month, besides your regular job, have you participated in any physical activities or sports, such as running, gymnastics, playing golf, gardening, or walking?" If the respondent answered in the affirmative, the question continued, "What type of physical activity or sport did you engage in most of the past month?" 75 different types of physical activity were grouped into eight categories, and frequency and duration were recorded.

In the total group, regardless of the amount of physical activity, people without physical activity reported a mean of 3.36 days with poor mental health ("mental health not good"). Individuals who reported any type of physical activity had 1.49 fewer days of distress, a 43% reduction. Individuals who had a history of depression reported poor mental health for nearly 11 days in the past month, physical activity reduced this time by a mean of 3.75 days, a 35% reduction. The association between physical activity was seen across the age range (people 18 years and older were surveyed), in both genders, in all ethnicities, and it was independent of household income.

For the first time, due to its size, this study also allowed a comparison of the effects of different types of exercise on psychological well-being. The strongest effects were found in popular team sports, followed by cycling, aerobic and fitness exercises, running or jogging, the optimal duration—regardless of the type of exercise—was between 30 and 60 min and the optimal frequency was three to five times per week. Similar ratios were found in people who had already suffered from depression. When mindfulness-based physical activities (yoga or tai chi) were analyzed separately, they had the strongest positive effects on mental health. I will return to mindfulness-based practices later in this chapter. Overall, the effects of physical activity on mental health were stronger than those of education level or household income. It is also interesting to note the finding that team sports had some of the strongest positive effects on mental health. This underscores the fact that, in addition to pure exercise, social activity also plays a significant role here [7].

One might object that finding an association does not mean that there is a causal relationship here, and likewise the causality could be reversed: better mental health results in people exercising more. However, the authors cite a number of reasons to believe that exercise does indeed lead to better mental health (and not the other way around). One important piece of evidence is the randomised controlled trials that have used physical activity as an intervention to treat various mental health conditions (depression, anxiety disorders, post-traumatic stress disorder). However, there are now also longitudinal studies (the above study is a cross-sectional study, i.e., the subjects were examined at a single time point, whereas a longitudinal study examines the same subject over time, i.e., at at least two time points) that demonstrate that physical activity prevents the onset of depression. The most convincing and largest such study was recently presented [8]. These researchers studied nearly 34,000 healthy adults with no previously known mental illness for a mean of eleven years. 7% of the subjects had developed depression at follow-up and 8.7% had developed an anxiety disorder. Subjects who reported no physical activity at baseline had a 44% higher risk of depression at follow-up than those who exercised one to two hours per week at baseline. However, no association with the risk of developing an anxiety disorder was found in this study. Although the authors acknowledge some methodological problems in the interpretation of such a large and long-term study, they conclude that even moderate sporting activity of one hour's duration could lead to 12% of cases of depression being prevented [8]. The positive effect increases with the duration of weekly activity, but it seems to reach a plateau at around four hours. The first hour of exercise has the greatest protective effects.

Another team of researchers meta-analyzed the question of whether physical activity protects against depression. In their analysis of 49 prospective studies with more than 266,000 subjects, they found that subjects who had a higher level of physical activity had a 17% lower risk of developing depression than those who exercised little. The finding was thus found for all age groups and geographical regions [9].

Finally, it should be noted that there is even clear evidence that not only aerobic endurance training but also strength training has antidepressant effects. This was the result of a recent meta-analysis of 33 randomized studies with a total of almost 1900 participants [10]. An antidepressant effect could also be demonstrated in those subjects who showed no increase in strength or muscle mass.

So, to sum up, there is overwhelming evidence for the positive health effects of physical activity. Compared to people who do not exercise or exercise very little, physically active people are less likely to develop cardiovascular diseases, strokes or diabetes mellitus, they live significantly longer and they enjoy better mental health. However, many of the authors working on the subject point out that the epidemic lack of physical activity that has gripped the entire world population is not just a problem for each individual. It is a problem that affects our societies as a whole. This again emphasizes that this is not about the "self-optimization" of the individual. It is about the attitude of a society towards its members and their health. Does it create the conditions of life—and here the *mental* conditions of life are meant in particular—that allow its members to live in health and well-being, or does it try to adapt people to increasingly adverse conditions of life that are no longer fair to human beings, e.g. through high-tech medicine? I will return to this important question at the end of this chapter.

Nutrition

We now also know for a fact that a plant-based diet low in animal fat and meat not only leads to better physical health, but is also associated with better mental performance and increased well-being. The incidence of overweight and obesity is reduced, as is that of diabetes mellitus and cardiovascular disease. Many cancers have also been shown to be influenced by dietary factors. Many types of cancer occur less frequently in populations with a predominantly plant-based diet than in societies where meat consumption is a sign of social affluence. Unsaturated fats from foods derived from animals also increase the oxidative stress of nerve cells, leading to their poorer energy supply and a breakdown of synaptic connections. There are now also studies showing that calorie restriction in general—i.e. regardless of the type of food consumed—leads to better physical health and increased cognitive performance.

One of the most important studies investigating the impact of diet on physical health was published in 2018 by a team of Spanish researchers in the prestigious New England Journal of Medicine (after the first version of the study, published in the same journal in 2013, was retracted by the authors due to methodological errors) [11]. In the study, with the acronym PREDIMED, approximately 7500 people between the ages of 55 and 80 years who had an increased cardiovascular risk but no cardiovascular event were randomly assigned to three groups. Two of the groups were instructed to eat according to the Mediterranean diet, and the third group was instructed to eat a low-fat diet. The group that was trained to eat the Mediterranean diet was given either additional olive oil or additional mixed nuts. The subjects were then followed for an average of just under five years and recorded whether a cardiovascular event (heart attack, stroke or death from such an event) occurred. By the end of the study, 96 and 83 events were recorded in the groups that ate a Mediterranean diet enriched with olive oil or nuts, respectively, and 109 events in the control group that had been trained to eat a low-fat diet. This may sound like only a small difference. However, the authors calculate a reduction in the risk of a cardiovascular event with a Mediterranean diet of about 30% [11].

Characteristics of the Mediterranean diet are a high proportion of olive oil, fruits, nuts, vegetables and cereals. Fish and poultry are consumed in moderate quantities, while at the same time the proportion of dairy products, red meat, processed meat and sweets is reduced. Wine, consumed in moderate amounts usually with meals, is also part of the classic Mediterranean diet.

Since as early as the 1960s, this dietary style, which was characteristic of Greece, especially Crete, and southern Italy, regions where olives are grown, has been associated with the longevity and good health of the populations there [12]. In recent years, with the epidemic increase in overweight, obesity, diabetes mellitus and other diet-associated diseases, research into the importance of our dietary style is now becoming increasingly important.

In the last 10–15 years or so, it has also become increasingly clear that nutrition also plays a very significant role in our cognitive performance and mental well-being. On the one hand, there is growing evidence that certain foods or dietary components—e.g. omega-3 fatty acids—protect or even improve brain function; on the other hand, we know that, for example, a dietary style rich in saturated (animal) fats not only increases the risk of cardiovascular and many other somatic diseases, but can also lead to mental and neurological dysfunction [13]. Omega-3 unsaturated fatty acids are found abundantly in fatty marine fish, certain vegetable oils (e.g., olive oil), and even nuts. It is also possible that it is the ratio between the proportion of omega-3 and omega-6 unsaturated fatty acids that accounts for the neuroprotective value of the Mediterranean diet [14]. In a sub-analysis of the Spanish PREDIMED study (see above), it was found that there tended to be less depression in the group that ate a Mediterranean diet enriched with nuts. This effect was also statistically significant in people suffering from type 2 diabetes mellitus [15].

Many such studies include too small a number of subjects to be able to derive statistically reliable statements from them. Therefore, in so-called meta-analyses, all studies available on a topic are examined and summarized using certain statistical methods. In this way, considerably larger samples are obtained. An Australian group of scientists examined all available studies on the relationship between dietary habits and depression. Although the number of these studies is still relatively small, they found a 15% reduced risk of depression in people who ate a diet rich in fruits and vegetables, whole grains, and fish [16]. In contrast, a statistical trend was found for an association between Western diets (high in meat, sugar, fat, energy-dense, and industrially processed foods) and an increased risk of depression. In a second such meta-analysis, Greek researchers examined the effects of a Mediterranean diet on the risk of several nervous system disorders, namely stroke, cognitive impairment, and depression [17]. They found that people who consistently ate a Mediterranean diet had about a 30% reduced risk of stroke or depression and a 40% reduced risk of cognitive impairment. Dementia risk was also reduced by a Mediterranean diet. Many of the positive effects on brain and mental health remain even if the Mediterranean diet is not consistently followed, only the protective effect against stroke could then no longer be demonstrated [17]. A Japanese research consortium was able to show that nutritional factors are also associated with the risk of suicide. Japan has one of the highest suicide rates in the world, so suicide prevention is particularly important there. They studied nearly 90,000 people in Japan over an average of almost nine years. In the process, they also recorded their dietary habits. They found that people whose diet were high in vegetables, fruits, potatoes, soy products, mushrooms, seaweed and fish had a reduced risk of suicide. Interestingly, the researchers found no associations between suicide risk and a traditional diet high in fish or a Western diet [18]. Canadian researchers also studied the relationship between mental health and diets rich in vegetables and fruits in their country [19]. Nearly 300,000 Canadians were asked about their consumption of vegetables and fruits on the one hand, and the presence of depression in the past 12 months in a brief diagnostic interview on the other. Factors such as smoking, household income, education level, physical activity and some more were taken into account in the statistical analysis. Greater consumption of vegetables and fruits resulted in up to 30% lower risk of depression and reduced experience of stress [19]. Finally, a recent meta-analysis of a total of 21 studies on the relationship between diet and depression risk concluded that a healthy diet reduced the risk of depression, while a Western-style diet increased the risk [20].

But how can these correlations be explained? We currently believe that it is most likely the animal fats that dominate the Western diet that have such significant negative effects on physical and mental health. Animal fats are particularly high in saturated fatty acids, the breakdown of which leads to a low-grade, chronic inflammatory response in the body. Such inflammatory processes have been plausibly implicated in numerous chronic diseases, including depression. For example, an association between the pro-inflammatory properties of diet and mortality has recently been demonstrated in two large population samples of more than 25,000 individuals [21].

Of course, many of these studies have the fundamental weakness that they only show associations and not causalities. This means that the effect could also be due to other factors that have not been recorded. For example, people who eat a more Mediterranean diet could generally be more health-conscious and exercise more. Or the causality is reversed: people who suffer less from stress and depression may have a healthier diet. Even if such alternative explanations are in principle possible in individual cases, the overall view of all available data shows that—similar to what was shown earlier in this chapter for physical activity—certain diets lead to better mental health and cognitive performance.

Also convincing in this regard are studies showing that maternal nutrition during pregnancy and in the early postnatal period (i.e. after birth) has an impact on the mental health of their children [22]. The large Norwegian Mother and Child Cohort Study recruited 23,000 mothers and their children, who were studied until the age of five. The mothers' diets were assessed during pregnancy, after 1.5 and after 3 years. The study showed an association between unhealthy diet during pregnancy and later emotional and behavioural problems in the children, even when adjusted for other influencing factors (e.g. smoking, age of parents, household income, etc.) [22]. Similar results were obtained in the Generation R Study conducted in Rotterdam. Here, the children of mothers who ate a more Mediterranean diet showed fewer problems with inattention and aggression than the children of mothers who ate a traditional Dutch diet (with a high proportion of meat, processed meat products, potatoes and margarine) [23].

A North American research team recently categorized a large number of foods according to their content of nutrients for which there is evidence that they have preventive or even therapeutic effects against depression. Such evidence exists for folic acid, iron, omega-3 unsaturated fatty acids, magnesium, potassium, selenium, thiamine, vitamin A, vitamins B6 and B12, vitamin C and zinc. Foods of animal and plant origin were evaluated separately. Among animal foods, mussels and oysters, various other seafood and organs such as liver had the highest nutrient content; among plants, leafy vegetables, lettuce, peppers and cruciferous vegetables (e.g. broccoli) were rated highest [24].

Finally, it is very significant that our diet even seems to influence our sensitivity to stress. Our Western diet seems to lead to an amplification of the physiological stress response, while a Mediterranean diet seems to favour stress resistance [25]. However, the very populations that eat the worst diets are also the ones that are exposed to the most social stress, namely those in the bottom third of the socioeconomic hierarchy (see Part 2 of the book for more on this). A team of researchers from the University of California at Davis examined more than 1300 Puerto Ricans living in Boston in the Boston Puerto Rican Health Study [26] for their health status in relation to their health behaviors. People who felt more stressed ate fewer fruits, vegetables, and proteins, but more salty snacks and sweets, and they exercised less. Concentrations of the stress hormone cortisol were elevated, as were insulin levels, and body mass index was also elevated in people who felt stressed. The latter two findings suggest an increased risk of developing diabetes mellitus. However, as is so often the case, these findings are associations, and the causal relationships can only be speculated [26].

As with physical activity, the importance of the way we eat goes beyond the individual. Eating is not only a fundamental human need that serves to absorb energy and thus to maintain the functions of life, it also connects us very essentially as a social community. Here, not only the question of what we eat is concerned, but also how and in whose society we eat. Thus, food and nutrition become questions of public health, which—even more so—can be sharpened into the question of where we want to develop as a social community. And for some years now, it has also become increasingly clear to us that questions of food affect our living conditions on earth, especially our climate. Agriculture—including animal husbandry here—is responsible for about 25% of all greenhouse gas emissions, it consumes about 70% of all fresh water, arable land covers about 40% of the Earth's land mass, and the over-fertilization of large arable areas has led to the poisoning of surface and groundwater [27]. The "EAT-Lancet Commission on healthy diets from sustainable food systems", a commission of the British scientific journal *Lancet*, has in a groundbreaking paper not only compiled all the data proving what constitutes a healthy diet (the statements very largely coincide with the statements in this chapter) [28]. They also show the significant impact this diet has on the environment and the future of our planet. In various scenarios developed by the group, this international consortium of scientists has examined the potential impact of sustainable dietary changes not only on population mortality, but also on the environmental changes that result, namely greenhouse gas emissions, consumption of arable land and fresh water, and consumption of nitrate and phosphorus as fertilizers [27]. The following four dietary styles, for which—as also presented in this chapter—positive effects on health are considered to be proven, were investigated.

Flexitarian: no processed meat, only small amounts of red meat (consumed once a week), moderate amounts of other foods of animal origin (poultry, fish, dairy), generous amounts of plant-based foods (fruits, vegetables, legumes, nuts).

Pescetarian: Meat is replaced two-thirds by fish and other seafood and one-third by fruits and vegetables.

Vegetarian: Meat is replaced two-thirds by legumes and one-third by fruits and vegetables.

Vegan: all food of animal origin is replaced two-thirds by legumes and one-third by fruits and vegetables.

In addition, the effects of replacing food of animal origin with food of plant origin in the global diet were investigated (in four different scenarios, between 25% and 100% replacement of animal food with plant food). Some of the results of the calculations are very impressive: completely eliminating food of animal origin would reduce mortality by more than 10%, especially in countries with high per capita incomes, and greenhouse gases would be reduced by more than 80%. However, fresh water consumption would also increase by 15%, and in middle and low per capita income countries the effects would be much smaller, as diets in these countries are much more plant-based anyway. Focusing diets globally on health aspects, i.e. switching to flexitarian, pescetarian, vegetarian or vegan diets, all also characterized by a low to complete absence of meat, would reduce mortality by 19% (flexitarian) to 22% (vegan) while also reducing greenhouse gas emissions by at least 54% (up to 87%). In the process, nitrate and phosphorus pollution would also be reduced by 20–25%, and less usable land and fresh water would be used [27]. Nutrition is therefore not an issue that concerns only each individual. It concerns us as a global community. If we eat a healthy diet, be it vegan or perhaps less strictly "just" flexitarian, we benefit as individuals, we are healthier, we lower our risk of cardiovascular disease and many cancers, we live longer, we are also better able to perceive and enjoy this better physical health because we have a lower risk of developing depression or even dementia. But the benefits go beyond that. We contribute to better living conditions on this planet, and in turn we create an environment that reflects positively on us as individuals—and on our children and grandchildren.

Meditation

"A new frontier in treatment of mental illnesses and other chronic conditions may not come from pharmaceutical companies, but from within, as mindfulness techniques gain traction." So begins a review article in one of the most prestigious medical journals [29]. Indeed, "mindfulness" has gained enormous attention in recent years also as a therapeutic technique in psychiatry, most recently when an internationally acclaimed study showed that the so-called "Mindfulness-Based Cognitive Therapy" (MBCT) may be as effective in reducing the risk of relapse in patients with recurrent depressive disorder as antidepressant pharmacotherapy [30]. However, mindfulness-based practices have been studied in recent years not only in terms of their effects on mental health. There are now also numerous studies on the influence of meditation techniques on physical dysfunctions.

Mindfulness has its origins in ancient Buddhist meditation techniques. The core of all mindfulness techniques is the intentional, non-judgmental directing of attention to the present moment with openness, curiosity and the willingness to accept the present as it is. Significant importance in introducing mindfulness techniques into the Western health care system is attributed to the American cardiologist Herbert Benson, who founded the Mind/Body Medical Institute at Massachusetts General Hospital in Boston. Subsequently, various therapeutic systems were developed from this, including Mindfulness-Based Stress Reduction (MBSR) according to Jon Kabat-Zinn and MBCT, but also transcendental meditation, yoga, Tai Chi and other techniques.

Western medicine has largely ignored mindfulness as a therapeutic and preventive technique until a few years ago. However, this has been changing over the last decade or so as evidence for its effectiveness in a wide variety of somatic and psychiatric disorders has begun to mount. Examples include the above-mentioned study on relapse prevention in recurrent depression, or a study—albeit much smaller—in older people with chronic sleep disorders. Here, a mindfulness-based therapy was significantly superior to an intervention to improve sleep hygiene [31]. Meditation techniques probably have not only a therapeutic, but above all a prophylactic value. Better control of attention as well as improved emotion regulation and self-awareness should reduce susceptibility to stress.

The fact that mindfulness as a medical technique is receiving more attention in Western (orthodox) medicine is certainly also due to the fact that efforts have been made in recent years to gain a scientific understanding of its mechanisms of action. Even in the most prestigious journals, current reviews can be found, e.g. on the "Neuroscience of Mindfulness Meditation" [32].

However, most authors agree that mindfulness needs to be further well evaluated, as many of the existing studies are too small and have methodological weaknesses. For example, a mindfulness technique cannot be investigated as easily in a randomized, double-blind study as a drug. Even blinding is not possible, and randomization is problematic because a mindfulness technique requires a high level of motivation and a lot of time to learn. People who are willing to engage in mindfulness will benefit most from it. It will be methodologically extraordinarily difficult to map this in a randomized trial. This interesting and inspiring review concludes, "Whether clinicians recommend mindfulness techniques to their patients depends not only on their availability, but also on their willingness to include these approaches in the evidence-based clinical armamentarium" [29].

Some of the researchers who themselves scientifically investigate the effects of meditation and mindfulness also warn against euphoria [32–34]. Many studies are celebrated in the media without meeting methodological quality criteria. Very few of the available studies have a control group, theoretical concepts on the mechanisms of action of meditation or mindfulness are not available, and undesirable effects have been almost completely ignored.

However, such effects do exist. Thus, even relatively short-term interventions could also lead to an increase in stress and depression and also to a reactivation of childhood traumas [33, 34]. Thus, the authors also raise the question of the reasons for the popularity that mindfulness has gained in recent years: "Does mindfulness appeal to the iPhone-distracted generation of millenials like psychoanalysis did to the repressed Victorians? Social scientists examining such questions are suggesting that mindfulness has become much more than an Eastern derived form of therapy; it is an ideology which purports to better everything and everyone, making a more compassionate, wise, peaceful and productive individual and society" [34]. Elsewhere, the authors write, "The replacement of orange-robed gurus by white-collared academics who speak of the benefits of 'being in the present moment' is a powerful social phenomenon, which is probably rooted in our culture's desire for quick fixes and its attraction to spiritual ideas divested of supernatural elements." They continue, "This grandiose expectation regarding the optimisation of human functioning through a meditation technique may be looked on as naïve; but it is also dangerous. [...] It does something else that we find worrying: it encourages a simplistic portrayal of the human mind and of our inner lives" [33]. It may be that the authors are right on this point: Mindfulness is probably too often misunderstood as "gymnastics for the soul." This is perhaps where the analogy to exercise and diet as ways to maintain physical and mental health should actually stop. Indeed, it is precisely a core message of this book that human beings do not—much less their psyches (or "souls"?)—function as deterministic mechanisms. Thus, it should be reiterated here that the ways of maintaining a healthy mind and body discussed in this chapter should not be understood as means of mechanical "self-optimization." Exercise and more conscious eating are dimensions that should remind humans again more closely of their embeddedness in a larger, planetary ecosystem, and mindfulness should be understood in this context as a spiritual way to deepen this connection. I will return to this in the concluding chapter.

I have shown in this chapter that each individual has considerable possibilities to maintain and even improve his or her physical and mental health. I have done this in such detail primarily to show that we are by no means just victims of our genes, which run a biological program that decides how we feel, what diseases we suffer from or how old we become. By consciously dealing with the foundations of our life, by shaping our environment and our everyday life, we can have an influence on all of this and significantly influence the course of our lives. But in order to do this consciously and not just follow another program, this time a social one, we need education. Educated people are not only more prosperous, they are also physically and mentally healthier and live longer than people who have no education. Perhaps education is even the most important factor of all for human well-being. It is education that makes it possible to shape the social environment in which people live. I will return to the central role of education in the last part of the book.

Having focused on the individual in this chapter, in the next chapters I will discuss how we as individuals can create social structures—in our working and living environments and in our education and health systems—that will enable us, our children and their descendants to have a future of health and well-being.

References

1. Rook A (1954) An investigation into the longevity of Cambridge sportsmen. BMJ 1:773–777
2. Lee IM, Shiroma EJ, Lobelo F et al (2012) Lancet physical activity series working group. Effect of physical inactivity on major non-communicable diseases worldwide: an analysis of burden of disease and life expectancy. Lancet 380:219–229
3. Wen CP, Wai JP, Tsai MK et al (2011) Minimum amount of physical activity for reduced mortality and extended life expectancy: a prospective cohort study. Lancet 378:1244–1253
4. World Health Organization, WHO (2010) Global recommendations on physical activity for health. https://www.who.int/dietphysicalactivity/publications/9789241599979/en/. Accessed on May 10th 2020
5. Schnohr P, Marott JL, Lange P, Jensen GB (2013) Longevity in male and female joggers: the Copenhagen city heart study. Am J Epidemiol 177:683–689
6. Schnohr P, O'Keefe JH, Marott JL et al (2015) Dose of jogging and long-term mortality: the Copenhagen city heart study. J Am Coll Cardiol 65:411–419
7. Chekroud SR, Gueorguieva R, Zheutlin AB et al (2018) Association between physical exercise and mental health in 1.2 million individuals in the USA between 2011 and 2015: a cross-sectional study. Lancet Psychiatry 5:739–746
8. Harvey SB, Øverland S, Hatch SL et al (2018) Exercise and the prevention of depression: results of the HUNT cohort study. Am J Psychiatry 175:28–36
9. Schuch FB, Vancampfort D, Firth J et al (2018) Physical activity and incident depression: a meta-analysis of prospective cohort studies. Am J Psychiatry 175:631–648
10. Gordon BR, McDowell CP, Hallgren M et al (2018) Association of efficacy of resistance exercise training with depressive symptoms: meta-analysis and meta-regression analysis of randomized clinical trials. JAMA Psychiatry 75:566–576

11. Estruch R, Ros E, Salas-Salvadó J et al, PREDIMED study investigators (2018) Primary prevention of cardiovascular disease with a mediterranean diet supplemented with extra-virgin olive oil or nuts. N Engl J Med 378:e34

12. Willett WC, Sacks F, Trichopoulou A et al (1995) Mediterranean diet pyramid: a cultural model for healthy eating. Am J Clin Nutr 61(6 Suppl):1402S–1406S

13. Gómez-Pinilla F (2008) Brain foods: the effects of nutrients on brain function. Nat Rev Neurosci 9:568–578

14. Loef M, Walach H (2013) The omega-6/omega-3 ratio and dementia or cognitive decline: a systematic review on human studies and biological evidence. J Nutr Gerontol Geriatr 32:1–23

15. Sánchez-Villegas A, Martínez-González MA, Estruch R et al (2013) Mediterranean dietary pattern and depression: the PREDIMED randomized trial. BMC Med 11:208

16. Lai JS, Hiles S, Bisquera A et al (2014) A systematic review and meta-analysis of dietary patterns and depression in community-dwelling adults. Am J Clin Nutr 99:181–197

17. Psaltopoulou T, Sergentanis TN, Panagiotakos DB et al (2013) Mediterranean diet, stroke, cognitive impairment, and depression: a meta-analysis. Ann Neurol 74:580–591

18. Nanri A, Mizoue T, Poudel-Tandukar K et al (2013) Japan public health center-based prospective study group. Dietary patterns and suicide in Japanese adults: the Japan public health center-based prospective study. Br J Psychiatry 203:422–427

19. McMartin SE, Jacka FN, Colman I (2013) The association between fruit and vegetable consumption and mental health disorders: evidence from five waves of a national survey of Canadians. Prev Med 56:225–230

20. Li Y, Lv MR, Wei YJ et al (2017) Dietary patterns and depression risk: a meta-analysis. Psychiatry Res 253:373–382

21. Garcia-Arellano A, Martínez-González MA, Ramallal R et al, SUN and PREDIMED study investigators (2019) Dietary inflammatory index and all-cause mortality in large cohorts: The SUN and PREDIMED studies. Clin Nutr 38:1221–1231

22. Jacka FN, Ystrom E, Brantsaeter AL et al (2013) Maternal and early postnatal nutrition and mental health of offspring by age 5 years: a prospective cohort study. J Am Acad Child Adolesc Psychiatry 52:1038–1047

23. Steenweg-de Graaff J, Tiemeier H, Steegers-Theunissen RP et al (2014) Maternal dietary patterns during pregnancy and child internalising and externalising problems. The Generation R Study. Clin Nutr 33:115–121

24. LaChance LR, Ramsey D (2018) Antidepressant foods: an evidence-based nutrient profiling system for depression. World J Psychiatry 8:97–104

25. Hodge A, Almeida OP, English DR et al (2013) Patterns of dietary intake and psychological distress in older Australians: benefits not just from a Mediterranean diet. Int Psychogeriatr 25:456–466

26. Laugero KD, Falcon LM, Tucker KL (2011) Relationship between perceived stress and dietary and activity patterns in older adults participating in the Boston Puerto Rican health study. Appetite 56:194–204

27. Springmann M, Wiebe K, Mason-D'Croz D et al (2018) Health and nutritional aspects of sustainable diet strategies and their association with environmental impacts: a global modelling analysis with country-level detail. Lancet Planet Health 2:e451–e461

28. Willett W, Rockström J, Loken B et al (2019) Food in the anthropocene: the EAT-Lancet commission on healthy diets from sustainable food systems. Lancet 393:447–492

29. Buchholz L (2015) Exploring the promise of mindfulness as medicine. JAMA 314:1327–1329

30. Kuyken W, Hayes R, Barrett B et al (2015) Effectiveness and cost-effectiveness of mindfulness-based cognitive therapy compared with maintenance antidepressant treatment in the prevention of depressive relapse or recurrence (PREVENT): a randomised controlled trial. Lancet 386:63–73

31. Black DS, O'Reilly GA, Olmstead R et al (2015) Mindfulness meditation and improvement in sleep quality and daytime impairment among older adults with sleep disturbances: a randomized clinical trial. JAMA Intern Med 175:494–501

32. Tang YY, Hölzel BK, Posner MI (2015) The neuroscience of mindfulness meditation. Nat Rev Neurosci 16:213–225

33. Farias M, Wikholm C (2016) Has the science of mindfulness lost its mind? BJPsych Bull 40:329–332

34. Farias M, Wikholm C, Delmonte R (2016) What is mindfulness-based therapy good for? Lancet Psychiatry 3:1012–1013

7

Man Influences His Biology: How World Views Shape the Future

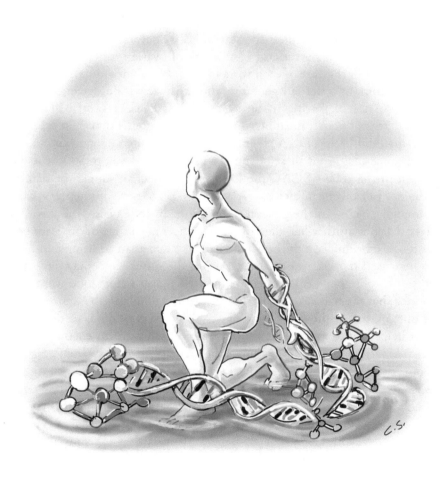

G. Gründer, *How Do We Want to Live?*, https://doi.org/10.1007/978-3-662-64225-2_7

Abstract Biomedical research suggests in its basic attitude that our physical and mental health and our risks of becoming physically or also mentally ill are determined by our biology, and here above all by our genes. But what is not true for physical illness is even less true for mental illness. We decide on our mental health and well-being to a large extent ourselves, once through our individual lifestyle, but much more through the design of our living environment. How strongly we are biologically determined and how we feel is a question of individual attitude, of "mindset", but also a question of the world view of our society.

When the very popular American actress, director and human rights activist Angelina Jolie had both breasts surgically removed in 2013, it made worldwide news. Jolie announced that she suffered from a genetic mutation that put her at a significantly increased risk of developing breast cancer. In an article in the New York Times, she stated, "My doctors estimated that I had an 87% risk of breast cancer and a 50% risk of ovarian cancer, although the risk is different in the case of each woman [...]. Only a fraction of breast cancers result from an inherited gene mutation. Those with a defect in BRCA1 have a 65% risk of getting it, on average" [1]. BRCA1 (and BRCA2) are tumor suppressor genes, meaning they code for proteins that help repair our genetic material DNA. DNA is constantly undergoing changes due to environmental factors. From these changes, a cancer can develop. So, if there is a mutation in the gene BRCA1, the DNA repair mechanism can be defective and the risk of cancer can increase. A woman's risk of developing breast cancer is estimated at 12% in the general population. In Jolie's case, there was also the fact that her mother had died of breast cancer at the age of 56, after being ill for ten years, which on the one hand can be taken as an additional indicator of an increased risk of breast cancer, but on the other hand may have motivated her to get genetically tested in the first place. Later, Jolie went on to announce that she had also had both ovaries and fallopian tubes removed. She went on to write in the New York Times, "For every woman reading this, I hope it helps you to know that you have options. I want to encourage every woman, especially if you have a family history of breast or ovarian cancer, to seek out the information and medical experts who can help you through this aspect of your life and to make your own informed choices" [1].

Who wouldn't opt for the removal of a not quite vital organ if they were told that they had an 87% chance of developing cancer in that very organ? Still, Jolie's decision was not at all as uncontroversial as it seems and as the numbers suggest. She writes that she had a choice, but her message is different: Genetics had just *not* given her a choice. The main criticism has been that Jolie's revelation could motivate other women to do the same, fuelling the trend towards mastectomies (the surgical removal of the mammary gland), which are not medically justified. In the U.S. in particular, oncologists and gynecologists report a veritable epidemic of mastectomies, especially when cancer has occurred in one breast. The other breast is then often removed as a precaution, even if there is no genetically increased risk. It is also often forgotten that a mutation of the BRCA1 or BRCA2 genes is found in only 5–10% of women with breast cancer and in 10–15% of women with ovarian cancer. In all other cases, there may also be a (still unknown) genetic basis, but here environmental factors may play at least as large or even larger a role. Thus, it is now undisputed that numerous environmental toxins and influences significantly affect the risk of most cancers. In the last chapter, I presented the extensive scientific evidence that today supports the importance of diet and exercise, including for the risk of developing many cancers. Jolie decided in 2015, two years after her first surgery, to have her ovaries and fallopian tubes removed as well. She received praise for this in the press and from doctors. The New York Times wrote, "Cancer experts said Tuesday that the actress and filmmaker Angelina Jolie Pitt was wise to have had her ovaries and fallopian tubes removed last week because she carries a genetic mutation, BRCA1, that significantly increases the risk of ovarian cancer, a disease so difficult to detect that it is often found only at an advanced, untreatable stage" [2]. This article also reiterated Jolie's choices, "They also said that Ms. Jolie Pitt's decision to discuss her own choices so frankly will encourage women in similar situations to consider their own options" [2]. It is likely that most people in comparable situations would have acted similarly; there wasn't really *a choice*. If the risk of contracting a disease that is virtually always fatal is 50% (and here we have to assume that the figures on which these risk estimates are based are really correct), if this disease is currently virtually impossible to detect at an early stage, and if, moreover, the organ from which the disease will potentially originate is not (any longer) vital, who would have acted differently?

However, the options may not always be so clear. Jolie was almost 38 years old at the time of her two surgeries and already had six children, so it's safe to assume that her family planning was complete. But what if a younger woman who has not yet had children gets genetic testing for a family history of breast and/or ovarian cancer and is found to carry a mutation in BRCA1 or BRCA2? At what point will she have surgery (she will be advised to do so before she turns 40)? What pressure will she be under to have children early? And she will wonder what the risk of being a gene carrier herself will be for her daughters. A young woman, 32, the mother of twin daughters, also describes this exact dilemma in the New York Times:

> Because I have, of course, passed the genes we now know are faulty to my children. Could they maybe be one of the lucky few? We won't be able to find out if they have inherited the mutation until they are 18 [because you may want to leave affected individuals to decide for themselves—as then adults—whether to get genetically tested—author's note]. On top of worrying what cancer will do to them should I have to go through it, I live every day now knowing they might have to go through it, too. And that's so much worse. I can handle cancer. I can handle anything. But my children? Have I sentenced them to pain, surgeries, chemotherapy or even death just by having them? I cannot bear the thought. [3]

The possible answer to this dilemma is also given in the very comprehensive coverage of the same newspaper: "It is also possible for women who are mutation carriers not to pass the gene on to their children by undergoing in vitro fertilization and having embryos tested for BRCA genes. Then only embryos free of mutations can be implanted" [4].

In vitro fertilisation (IVF), also known more simply as "artificial insemination", has also long been a routine method in Germany when a couple cannot conceive naturally. Preimplantation genetic diagnosis (PGD), as recommended in the article, is used to decide whether an embryo "created" by IVF should be implanted into the mother's uterus. PGD is allowed in most European countries (Catholic Italy is an exception), but usually only to prevent hereditary diseases. In the USA, however, PGD is already regularly used to select the desired sex of the embryo ("social sexing"), i.e. only embryos of the desired sex are implanted into the uterus. Over the years, PGD has experienced an expansion of indications. It is increasingly being used to detect diseases that previously could only be detected by prenatal diagnostics (i.e. in the already growing fetus), which can help to avoid abortions. In 1992, it was first reported that a healthy baby girl was born to genetically affected parents in the UK after PGD had ruled out the serious hereditary disease cystic fibrosis [5]. The value of PGD in such monogenically inherited, severe diseases, which always lead to premature death, is undisputed, even taking into account that people born with cystic fibrosis today live to forty years of age due to improved treatment options, whereas in the past they regularly died in childhood or adolescence.

However, mutations in the BRCA1 or BRCA2 gene do not necessarily lead to cancer, they do, as illustrated by the example, increase the risk, albeit very significantly in this case. For many people, the PGD route proposed in the

New York Times article, and the "selection" it entails, may be acceptable in light of the serious, often fatal, diseases that usually involve a great deal of suffering. However, the dilemmas this raises are obvious. Most of the diseases that kill people in industrialized societies today have a polygenetic basis. This means that there are several, often dozens, of genes that influence the risk of contracting a particular disease. Environmental influences are at least as important, and it is the interaction of genes and environment that ultimately determine overall risk. This is also true for most cancers. The exact risk for a particular disease will never be determined because it is influenced by environmental factors. From this perspective, a statement like Angelina Jolie made—"an 87% risk of breast cancer and a 50% risk of ovarian cancer"—is a gross oversimplification. There can be no such exactness. But if there were: at what risk of disease is selection—or "screening"—of an embryo justifiable? 50%? That still seems high. 20%? For many people, that might be a risk they could live with, especially if good treatment options were available in the event of a disease. But many surely wish to live without any worry of ever developing cancer. Can the vision of modern biomedicine offer that?

There are definitely also genetic factors that very significantly influence our risk of whether we will develop a psychiatric illness. For example, the genetic factors that influence the risk of developing Alzheimer's dementia are relatively well understood. Alzheimer's dementia is the most common form of dementia. More than 90% of cases occur sporadically and after the age of 65. They are called "sporadic" not because they occur rarely, but because they are not familial, meaning they can occur in previously unaffected families. For the rare, so-called "familial" (because they occur in families) cases, single gene mutations are known to drastically increase the risk of the disease and often cause affected individuals to become ill well before the age of 65. This is why they are also referred to as "presenile" dementias. However, it has also been known since the 1990s that the gene for apolipoprotein E (ApoE for short) influences our risk of developing Alzheimer's dementia.

ApoE is a protein that plays a central role in the transport and metabolism of fats and cholesterol [6]. The gene is present in three variants: ApoE ε2, ApoE ε3, and ApoE ε4. Since there are always two copies ("alleles") of each gene in humans, there are six different possible combinations in which the two alleles can be present in an individual human (ε2/ε2; ε2/ε3; ε3/ε3; ε2/ε4; ε3/ε4; ε4/ε4). If a person has two identical copies of a gene, they are said to be "homozygous" for that gene (i.e., ε4/ε4, for example). If the two alleles are not identical, he is "heterozygous" (e.g. ε2/ε3). The most common "normal" allele is ApoE ε3, and its frequency in the population is 77%, the frequency of ApoE ε4 is 15%, and the least common is ApoE ε2 at about 8%. If a person has one ApoE ε4 allele, his risk of developing Alzheimer's dementia triples (compared to a person with two ApoE ε3 alleles). If he is a homozygous ApoE ε4 carrier, his risk of disease is even 15-fold increased compared to the homozygous ApoE ε3 carrier [6, 7]. Conversely, the ApoE ε2 allele apparently has a protective effect; carriers of this allele have a lower risk of developing Alzheimer's dementia compared to a homozygous ApoE ε3 allele carrier [8].

These figures have not only academic significance. In the collective described by the scientists who first reported the significance of ApoE as a risk factor, people without an ApoE ε4 allele developed Alzheimer's dementia at a mean age of 84 years ("mean" here means that 50% of the people developed the disease at this age). If they carried an ApoE ε4 allele, the age dropped to 76 years, and homozygous ApoE ε4 carriers had 50% disease by age 68. Ten years later, 90% of this group had the disease [7]. On the other hand, homozygous ApoE ε4 carriers are not so common that one could infer that AD would suddenly become threateningly common beyond the age of 65. From an allele frequency of 15% in the general population, a frequency of 2% of homozygous ApoE ε4 carriers is calculated, and another 13% of the population is heterozygous for the ApoE ε4 allele. By far the majority of the population, 60%, are homozygous ApoE ε3 carriers. However, even for those who carry a risk allele, this does not mean that they will necessarily develop dementia. In Chaps. 5 and 6 we saw that the risk of developing dementia can be influenced very significantly.

Alzheimer's dementia is already an example of a disease that is relatively strongly genetically determined. For most psychiatric diseases, there are still no known genes that have a strong effect on the risk of the disease—despite decades of efforts costing billions. For schizophrenia (and certain severe forms of autism), for example, there are genetic variants (so-called "copy number variations", CMVs) that greatly increase the risk of disease. These variants are very rare, however, and no genetic abnormalities are found in most people with the disease. Instead, in recent years, through large-scale studies of tens of thousands of patients and healthy volunteers, a variety of risk genes have been identified that slightly increase the risk of developing schizophrenia. For example, in 2014, a very large international group of scientists reported in the prestigious journal *Nature* that from the studies of the genomes of 37,000 people suffering from schizophrenia and 113,000 healthy control subjects, they found 108 risk genes that increased the risk of disease, but with only a small effect [9]. The number of identified risk genes is constantly increasing, and now exceeds 200, from which a so-called "polygenic risk score" is calculated. After decades of searching for "genes for schizophrenia" were not crowned with success, the calculation of the individual risk of disease from the knowledge of the entire genome is now celebrated as a breakthrough. But what do we actually know about the genetic conditionality of this disease, which has always been a mystery, if we associate the risk of contracting it with several hundred risk genes? The American psychiatrist Kenneth Kendler, an expert on the genetics of psychiatric disorders, had already considered in 2005 that the concept according to which the expression of a specific gene "preforms" a certain trait or even a defined disease in a simple, direct and strong way had failed. He wrote: "The impact of individual genes on risk for psychiatric illness is small, often nonspecific, and embedded in complex causal pathways. The phrase 'a gene for' and the preformationist concept of gene action that underlies it are inappropriate for psychiatric disorders" [10].

Until a few years ago, it was actually believed that the risk of even severe, supposedly strictly biological, mental illness was the same across cultures and social contexts. For example, it was considered a well-established scientific fact that the lifetime prevalence, i.e., the risk of developing a particular disorder over a lifetime, for schizophrenia was 1% across countries and cultures. However, this is not so. It has long been known that people who live in cities have a higher risk of developing schizophrenia [11]. Recently, this has been explained by the fact that people who have a higher genetic risk of developing the disease are more likely to seek out an urban environment [12, 13]. However, this probably greatly underestimates the role of the living environment. A very recent Danish study investigated how strongly the risk of developing schizophrenia is influenced by the extent to which one spends one's childhood in a natural, "green" environment. To this end, they categorised the vegetation of Denmark on the basis of satellite photographs and related the vegetation index thus obtained to the risk of developing the illness. The results are remarkable: people who had spent their childhood in regions with the highest index (i.e. in very rural regions) had only half the risk of developing schizophrenia as people who had spent their childhood in regions with the lowest index (i.e. in metropolitan city centres without greenery). A large group of people also had their polygenetic risk score determined, and again the results were significant: the effect of polygenetic risk score on schizophrenia risk was significantly smaller than the effect of childhood environment. Even individuals with the highest risk score had only about a 25% increased risk of disease [14].

In a major project funded by the European Union, an international consortium of psychiatric researchers recently looked at the incidences (remember: this is the number of new cases in a defined observation period) of schizophrenic and affective psychoses. There had been no studies on this subject since the 1980s. The study examined 17 catchment areas, some of them very different, in five European countries (England, France, Italy, the Netherlands, Spain) and Brazil [13]. The catchment areas varied greatly, ranging from very rural regions (Cuenca, Spain, with 11 inhabitants per km^2) to megacities (Paris, 33,260 inhabitants per km^2). The researchers found a huge variance in first-episode disease rates. While in Santiago, Spain, it was 6.3 new cases per 100,000 person-years, in South London a tenfold higher first episode rate was found, at 61.4 per 100,000 person-years. This is surely due to the high numbers of migrants and other members of minority groups living in particularly high numbers in South London, who are at increased risk of contracting the disease. When corrected for this factor, the rate of first illness nevertheless remains highly variable. It is about eight times higher in Paris and South London than in Santiago. The study initially confirmed the findings of previous research on a significantly increased risk of psychosis among ethnic minorities and among (younger) men. However, the study was able to document other interesting findings. For example, incidences in southern Europe were in some cases considerably lower than in northern Europe, but no correlation with latitude could be found. Incidence rates were also found to be lower in regions where residents lived in residential properties. This factor is not only an indicator of the socio-economic conditions of a society, but also of social stability and cohesion. The last finding in particular is very significant, as it could explain the lower morbidity rates in southern European countries, where family and social networks are even more important than in central and northern European countries.

The nonspecific way in which genes influence the risk of developing psychiatric disorders was again made particularly clear when a large consortium of researchers reported at the end of 2018 that alcohol dependence shares its genetic basis with 17 other psychiatric disorders, including schizophrenia, depression and attention deficit hyperactivity disorder [15]. But if the effects of certain gene variants are so nonspecific, what does it tell us if we carry five, ten, or even three dozen of these risk variants in our genes? Don't we know anyway—and doesn't our everyday experience already show us this—that we all, every single person, carry a high risk of developing mental illness? On the other hand, even people who carry one of the rare Copy Number Variations, which are associated with a greatly increased risk of schizophrenia, will not fall ill with absolute certainty. The same applies to the healthy identical twins of people suffering from schizophrenia. Here, the diseased and the non-diseased person have the same genetic make-up, and it can only be environmental conditions in the broadest sense that cause one twin to become ill and the other to remain healthy.

There are still scientists who believe in a strict genetic conditionality of mental disorders. They argue that we only need to know enough about the precise genetic mechanisms that lead to the disorder. Once we understand how the biochemical machinery of the brain is regulated by genes, it will eventually be possible to use genetic diagnostics to determine the individual risk of disease. However, the prospects for therapeutic approaches to be derived from this sound appropriately vague: "The systematic elucidation of biological causes through genetic and subsequent functional investigations will be the starting point for the development of new drug strategies" [16]. This statement from a scientific article published in 2019 could have appeared like this twenty years earlier, in 1999. Unfortunately, it is not one iota more concrete today. Decades of genetic research have not brought us even close to any therapy for any psychiatric disease.

For some years now, hope has therefore been placed in the relatively new field of epigenetics. It teaches us that our genome, as each of us inherits it from our parents, is not a static matrix whose information is simply read and translated into proteins. The base sequence that determines the information of our DNA is—if we disregard sporadic mutations, i.e. spontaneously occurring changes—static and unchangeable. But this is only half the truth. Whether a gene is read and its information then leads to the synthesis of a protein (this is referred to as gene expression) is decided by certain markers on the DNA or on the proteins (so-called histones), with the help of which the DNA is packed into a very small space. How these markers in turn behave biologically is essentially controlled by environmental influences. Epigenetics is therefore readily understood as a science that integrates genetic and environmental influences. "Epi" genetic (epi, Greek, = over) influences go beyond genetic influences or regulate the function of genes without altering the genetic information itself. A well-studied example of the importance of epigenetics is the regulation of the glucocorticoid receptor. Glucocorticoids—the best known of this group of hormones is cortisol—are important molecules in hormonal stress regulation. Stress hormones such as cortisol exert their effect via precisely this glucocorticoid receptor. The number of these receptors in the brain, in turn, significantly influences the sensitivity to stress—a high density of the receptor is associated with a lower sensitivity to stress and vice versa. Whether the gene for the glucocorticoid receptor is now expressed and thus many of these receptors are present in our brain is largely determined by early childhood experiences. Negative early childhood experiences, e.g. separation from the mother, lead to a reduced expression of the gene via certain changes in the DNA (in technical jargon: "methylation" of the promoter of the glucocorticoid receptor gene). This results in a reduced number of glucocorticoid receptors in the developing brain, leading to increased stress reactivity that persists into adulthood. Conversely, it has been shown in rats that particularly intense affection from rat mothers towards young rats results in reduced methylation, which leads to improved robustness to stress in adulthood via increased expression of glucocorticoid receptors. Such associations have also been shown in humans. People who had taken their own lives and who had been abused or mistreated in childhood were found to have higher DNA methylation and consequently a reduced number of glucocorticoid receptors than suicide victims who had not been known to have been abused [17]. Many other such epigenetic changes as a result of traumatic childhood experiences are now known, demonstrating that early childhood biography leaves deep marks on our biology. However, it is by no means the case that these traces have to be negative; the opposite is also true. As the example of the sheltered rats shows, positive early childhood experiences can lead to reaction patterns and behaviour that have a significant positive influence on the rest of life. Child abuse and maltreatment are among the most significant risk factors for the development of psychiatric illness in adults. Psychosocial interventions that reduce or eliminate negative early childhood experiences are therefore important preventive measures to reduce the incidence of psychiatric illness. In a study of 188 mothers with poor psychosocial backgrounds and correspondingly increased risk for abuse of their children, half of the mothers were followed by nurses as part of a psychosocial program; the other half of the mothers represented the control group without such an intervention. The mothers' offspring had the extent to which their DNA was methylated (as a sign of early childhood stress) measured at age 27. It was found that both early childhood abuse (a negative) and participation in the psychosocial prevention program (a positive) had an effect on DNA methylation [18]. More and more studies suggest that early childhood environment and also psychosocial status have considerable influence on the epigenetic regulation of our genome. It is now also known that such epigenetic changes in our DNA induced by environmental factors can also be passed down through generations [19]. These findings put the deterministic importance of our genes for our fate into perspective. Epigenetic changes are also not irreversible. They can be altered by both psychotherapy and pharmacotherapy.

A very remarkable study recently published by a team of psychologists from Stanford University in California shows that the individual "mind" can influence our bodily functions to a considerable extent, and that this influence can even be more significant than the effect of a genetic variant. We have already seen in Chap. 3 how significantly expectancy can influence the effect of drug therapy. When the effect is positive, we know it as the placebo effect, and when the expectation has a negative effect (e.g. side effects), we know it as the nocebo effect. The American researchers investigated what physiological effects would occur in healthy subjects simply by *knowing* their genotype (i.e. genetic pattern) with regard to certain bodily functions [20]. To this end, they conducted two experiments on the role of risk genes for obesity (see also Chap. 2). In the first, they determined the genotype of a gene that influences endurance performance in 116 subjects. People with a certain variant of the gene are more efficient than those with another variant, and this in turn reduces their risk of obesity. After testing, all subjects underwent a performance test on a treadmill. Only then were they told whether they were carriers of the "high-risk" variant or the "protective" variant of the gene. However, the result communicated did not necessarily correspond to the true result of the test. That is, some of the subjects who actually belonged to the high-risk group were told that they had the protective genotype, and conversely, some of the subjects who actually had the protective variant were told that the high-risk variant had been found in them. Immediately after the clarification, they were subjected to a second test on the treadmill, before they were naturally informed of the true conditions afterwards. The performance of subjects who had been told before the second run that they had the protective genotype did not change. However, subjects who had been told they had the high-risk genetic variant performed significantly worse on the second test in several performance parameters. The most interesting finding, however, was that the effect of being told about a particular genotype on performance was greater than the effect of the true genotype on several measures! This means that the expectation effect had a stronger effect on physiology than the gene, or, to put it more succinctly: "Mind over Matter"!

In order to further substantiate their findings, the Stanford scientists conducted a second, similar experiment: This time, 107 healthy volunteers were characterized with regard to a gene that is considered one of the most significant risk genes for the development of obesity. Subjects with the high-risk variant are less quickly satiated; this is also reflected physiologically in a reduced release of intestinal peptides that signal a feeling of satiety to the body. When subjects with this genetic variant are shown images of food, they respond with greater activation in specific brain regions that signal appetite and reward. After a standardized meal, the subjective feeling of satiety and the release of the satiety peptide "glucagon-like peptide 1" (GLP-1) were measured in all subjects. Then, again regardless of their "true" genotype, half of the subjects were informed that they were carriers of the high-risk variant of the gene, and the other half were informed that they were carriers of the "protective" variant. At a second meal, one week later, again completely standardized for composition and energy content, they again measured subjective satiety and release of the peptide. The results were even more impressive than in the first experiment. Regardless of their "true" genetic makeup, subjects who believed they were genetically "protected" had a significantly greater release of the hormone GLT-1 after eating the same meal and, associated with this, a much greater feeling of satiety than the subjects who had been told they were carriers of the risk gene. And in this second experiment, the effects of the "told" genotype, i.e., the expectation, were also significantly greater than those of the "true" genotype [20].

Many questions follow here. What does it mean when more and more people are gaining more and more information about their genes? One in 25 Americans, or 4% of the population, now obtains such personalized information, and their numbers are rising rapidly. In 2017, more Americans had themselves genetically tested for any disease risk than in all previous years combined [21]. In discussing genes that influence our risk for breast cancer or Alzheimer's disease, we have seen that this influence can be substantial. In the last chapter, however, we also noted that the risk of dementia is not set in stone, but can be influenced—that is, lowered (!)—to a quite significant degree by lifestyle factors. And the studies from Stanford described here show that the effects of genes with a small effect can be insignificant compared to expectation, placebo or nocebo effects.

The example of weight regulation in particular shows the different perspectives from which the problem of obesity can be viewed. Of course, the interaction between genes and environmental factors also regulates our energy metabolism and thus ultimately whether we are underweight, normal weight or overweight. The importance of environmental factors in this context is shown by the enormous increase in the incidence of overweight and obesity worldwide in recent decades. This topic has been discussed in detail in Chap. 2. This subject is also an excellent example of how medical research influences the perception of the problem. However, perception also controls how we all deal with it. So says the introduction to a major review in the prestigious journal *Lancet Diabetes Endocrinology*:

Genome-wide association studies (GWAS) for BMI, waist-to-hip ratio, and other adiposity traits have identified more than 300 single nucleotide polymorphisms (SNPs; [single nucleotide polymorphism: a variant in our genome that makes people different from one another—author's note]). While there is reason to hope that these discoveries will eventually lead to new preventive and therapeutic agents for obesity, this will take time because such developments require detailed mechanistic understanding of how an SNP affects phenotype (and this information is largely unavailable) [22].

In this paper, the genetic contribution (called heritability) to obesity is reported to be 40–70%, and "therapeutics for obesity" are—of course—drugs. In the same issue of the journal, it says:

> Healthy lifestyle choices are the foundation of obesity treatment. However, weight loss can lead to physiological adaptations that promote weight regain. As a result, lifestyle treatment alone typically produces only modest weight loss that is difficult to sustain. In other metabolic diseases, pharmacotherapy is an accepted adjunct to lifestyle [23].

After all, the authors of these papers state that lifestyle changes are the basis of obesity treatment, only to point out that these measures will not be sufficient. Again, we have to ask ourselves whether drug therapy is the right strategy to address the global obesity pandemic. We know that it was and is primarily changes in our living conditions that have caused the incidence of overweight and obesity to rise dramatically in recent decades. And we also know that as the incidence of overweight increases, so does the risk of many other diseases, and these include not only diabetes, but also diseases that we are fighting with the tools of high-tech medicine, for example: cancer. And further, we know that obesity and depression are associated with each other, they even seem to be two sides of the same coin in many cases (see also Chap. 2). Before we intervene in our biology with the means of modern high-performance medicine, should we not first ask ourselves how we can make our environment and our lifestyle more life-friendly again?

I would like to cite one more random example—thousands of them could easily be found—from the medical literature that shows how the supposedly so value-free science shapes our perception of ourselves. Countless studies over the past years and decades suggest that chronic stress leads to a mild inflammatory response in the body. This can be demonstrated not only in animal studies, but in humans as well. Animals, for example rats, then also show characteristics in neurobiology and behavior similar to those observed in humans in the context of depression. In fact, many studies in humans with depression suggest that similar mechanisms are at work here. Apparently, stress triggers certain immunological responses that lead to malaise and dejection, and then ultimately depression, in animals as well as humans. A very characteristic current scientific paper summarizes the typical approach to the problem thus:

> Depression is a prime contributor to global disease burden with 300 million affected patients worldwide. The persistent lack of progress with regards to

pharmacotherapy stands in stark contrast to the pandemic magnitude of the disease. Alterations of inflammatory pathways in depressed patients, including altered circulating pro-inflammatory cytokines, have been put forward as a potential pathophysiological mechanism. The P2X7 receptor (P2X7R) plays an important role regulating the release of interleukin-1β and other cytokines. Comprehensive investigation of the P2X7R Gln460Arg missense mutation (rs2230912), which has been associated with major depression and bipolar disorder, has substantially contributed to validate P2X7R as a potential genetic risk factor. We propose that P2X7R is a putative target with good prospects for therapeutic intervention in depressive disorders [24].

What is formulated here in typical medical jargon can also be expressed more simply as follows: "Depression is accompanied by a mild, chronic inflammatory reaction (perhaps it is even its consequence). So we treat depression by inhibiting the inflammatory response". There is no question that biological processes play a significant role in the development of depression. But are we going to cope with the pandemic of 300 million people affected by it by developing substances that influence the immune response to stress? Is it not at least as sensible to ask how and why our living conditions have changed in such a way that more and more people suffer from changes in the function of their immune system—among numerous other physical dysfunctions—and this then ultimately leads to depression? It is good and important that we explore the biological basis of our behaviour. We've accumulated a tremendous amount of knowledge over the past few decades about what changes in the body—and especially the brain—are associated with depression. But that is precisely the crucial formulation: *they accompany depression,* but we do not know (as the formulations from the publication cited above suggest) whether they are the *cause of the* depression. Similarly, it is conceivable that the dysfunction of the P2X7R receptor, identified as "a potential target for therapeutic intervention in depressive disorders," is a *consequence of* depression. There are undoubtedly well known physical causes of depression. For example, when people with certain diseases such as multiple sclerosis (MS) are treated with beta-interferon, many of those so treated develop depression. Interferon interferes in a significant way with the function of the immune system, and just such observations suggest that the function of the immune system in certain cases plays an important role in our mental state. However, this does not mean that it is always impaired immune function that underlies depression. In fact, in most cases it may be the other way around, or, more plausibly, it may be two sides of a phenomenon that we artificially separate, even though it is impossible to separate. We construct a separation of body and mind, suggesting that there is a causal conditionality here. Modern biomedicine— and especially biological psychiatry—regards the mind as an epiphenomenon of bodily processes. If this were so, we would indeed be at the mercy of the dictates of our genes—we would literally have no choice.

In fact, the Stanford University study shows that we have many more choices than modern gene-centered biomedicine suggests. We are not strictly determined by our genes! We have discussed in Chap. 6 numerous examples of the influence our individual lifestyles have on our physical and mental health. However, we can actually shape our living environment in such a way that we not only experience greater psychological well-being in it, but also experience our body as healthier again. In doing so, we will also blur the lines between mind and body that our understanding of ourselves has made ever sharper.

In her world-famous "Counterclockwise" study, which she conducted in the fall of 1981, Harvard psychologist Ellen Langer impressively demonstrated how personal attitudes (the "mindset"; she also wrote a book with this title) can influence even such supposedly strongly biologically determined processes as aging [25]. Langer and her team recruited two groups of eight elderly men each, who were in their late seventies or early eighties. Both groups were then isolated in specially prepared rooms for a week. These rooms provided an exact replica of the subjects' environment as it had been twenty years earlier, in 1959. Music from that year was played, and films shown were from 1959, as were the newspapers and books provided. One group (the experimental group) of old people were now instructed to behave exactly as they had twenty years earlier. They were asked to write a short autobiography as if they were current in 1959, and to bring photographs that showed them in 1959. Each interview was to be conducted in the present tense, as if it had actually taken place in 1959. The control group lived one week later under exactly the same spatial conditions. However, this group was to write a resume in the past tense, and the pictures its members brought showed them in 1981. In addition, they were instructed to reminisce about 1959 but to talk about it in the past tense. Langer writes about the instructions to the members of the experimental group in her book:

> Therefore, we're going to a very beautiful retreat where we will live as *if* it were 1959. Obviously, that means no one can discuss anything that happened after September 1959. It is your job to help each other do this. It is a difficult task, since we are not asking you to 'act as if it is 1959' but to let yourself be just who you were in 1959. We have good reason to believe that if you are successful at this, you also will feel as well as you did in 1959 [25].

The results of the study were remarkable, and they attracted so much international attention that they were worthy of a major story in the New York Times Magazine as late as 2014: "What if age is nothing but a mindset?" [26]. Both groups of men improved in many of the parameters used to track their health. After just one week, they heard better, they had better memory, and they had gained weight. The experimental group gained joint mobility and finger length as symptoms of arthritis improved. 63% of the subjects in the experimental group and 44% in the control group improved their intelligence quotient. Height increased, and posture and stance improved. Finally, uninvolved individuals who were not informed of the study objective were asked to rate photographs of the study participants taken at the end of the week in terms of the age of the individuals pictured. After one week, the participants in the experimental group were not only assessed as being significantly younger than before the start of the retreat, but also younger than the individuals in the control group.

In her book, Ellen Langer explores the extent to which the mind can influence the body. She writes, "If the mind were in a truly healthy place, the body would be quite the same, and we could change our physical health by changing our minds" [25]. Langer has a very individual perspective on this: she postulates that individuals can influence their personal health through their minds. In this book, however, I go beyond this perspective. Especially in this chapter and then in the third part of the book, I show that man is only in (small?) part a victim of his genes, which unfold a genetic program. He is above all a shaper of his living environment, and in shaping his living environment he actually has a choice about his health, and health here—in line with the WHO definition—is understood not only as the absence of disease or infirmity, but a state of complete physical, mental and social well-being [27]. Do we see ourselves as biological machines, albeit incredibly complex ones, which we only need to understand sufficiently well in order to then control them in such a way that they can cope with even the most adverse living conditions in the future? Once we have understood how our genes also control our psychological state, will we in future optimise our genome—for example through pre-implantation diagnostics—in such a way that our offspring are more resilient to hostile living, working and environmental conditions? Will we improve our ability to cope with these conditions through a cocktail of tailor-made drugs adapted to our individual biology?

Over the last few decades, we have evolved into this reductionist view of humanity, and it seems that it has not served us well. While our physical health has improved, often with the help of numerous medications, and we are living longer, our mental health has obviously deteriorated significantly.

More and more people, especially young people, feel overwhelmed by the demands of an increasingly complex work environment, and social relationships are being replaced by 'social networks'. We saw in Chap. 3 that the consumption of antidepressants in Germany has doubled in the last 15 years. In the US, 12% of people over the age of 12 take an antidepressant, most of them for five years or even longer. Psychiatric research seems to be fighting a desperate defensive battle: While more and more details are being amassed about how our brains work, more and more subtle biological dysfunctions are being found in psychiatric disorders, it remains completely unclear how psychological experience is coupled to or arises from brain function. The enormous scientific findings of brain research in recent decades hardly reach the patient. So confessed Tom Insel, the then director of the American Institutes of Mental Health (NIMH; the main agency for psychiatric research and its funding in the US) after his move to Google in 2015:

> I spent 13 years at NIMH really pushing on the neuroscience and genetics of mental disorders, and when I look back on that I realize that while I think I succeeded at getting lots of really cool papers published by cool scientists at fairly large costs—I think $20 billion—I don't think we moved the needle in reducing suicide, reducing hospitalizations, improving recovery for the tens of millions of people who have mental illness. I hold myself accountable for that [28].

Neurobiology and genetics are certainly important determinants of mental disorders, possibly as important as cancer. But they do not determine us. Ellen Langer, in her Counterclockwise study, suggested the profound ways in which an individual's mindset can influence his or her body.

The central thesis of this book is that man, through his individual psychological experience, can not only determine his own personal destiny—and thus his psychological and physical well-being. He can also shape his social environment so that the individuals who make up a society have a better life. And it is not only the individual's attitude that significantly influences his destiny. Today, it is probably much more the mindset of an entire society that determines the direction in which it develops, and with it the direction of the individuals who make up that society. So we are not just talking about a "mindset" of the individual, but the "mindset" of a whole social community. In hierarchically organized biological systems, the "higher", more complex level of the hierarchy has a causal effect on the "lower" levels. Already in Chap. 4 we learned—in connection with the discussion of placebo and nocebo effects—that the American psychologist Donald T. Campbell coined the term "downward causation". In a well-received article ("Downward Causality in Hierarchically Organized Biological Systems") he wrote already in 1974:

> The laws of the higher-level [...] system determine in part the distribution of lower-level events and substances. Description of an intermediate-level phenomenon is not completed by describing its possibility and implementation in lower-level terms. Its presence, prevalence, or distribution (all necessary for a complete explanation of biological phenomena) will often require reference to laws of a higher level of organization as well. [...] All processes at the lower levels of a hierarchy are restrained by and act in conformity to the laws of the higher levels [29].

This principle is fundamentally opposed to the central principle of reductionism: "All processes at the higher levels are restrained by and act in conformity to the laws of the lower levels, including the levels of subatomic physics" [29]. No one will seriously question this principle. Complex brain function is inconceivable without the subtle interplay of billions of neurons, and complex mental experience is inconceivable without an intact brain. This becomes very clear at the latest when dementia deprives us of our highest brain functions. But can consciousness and individual psychological experience be explained by the laws of neurophysiology alone (or even by the laws of particle physics)? No one has yet been able to explain in terms of physics, biology, or chemistry how thoughts arise. Conversely, I have given examples in this chapter of how the power of "mind" affects our physiology. And our social systems affect, in significant ways, how the individuals who make up those social systems function and interact with each other. I will return to this in Chap. 8.

In his important book "Man's search for meaning" (German: "Trotzdem Ja zum Leben sagen"), the Viennese psychiatrist Viktor Frankl laid down the counter-project to the model of modern biomedicine:

> By the same token, every human being has the freedom to change at any instant. Therefore, we can predict his future only within the large framework of a statistical survey referring to a whole group; the individual personality, however, remains essentially unpredictable. The basis for any predictions would be represented by biological, psychological or sociological conditions. Yet one of the main features of human existence is the capacity to rise above such conditions, to grow beyond them. Man is capable of changing the world for the better if possible, and of changing himself for the better if necessary [30].

Can words better describe the situation of man in a world in which the individual in his thinking, feeling and acting is only a biological mechanism mediating between on the one hand genetic and biological, on the other hand environmental factors, than these sentences written more than 50 years ago?

What Frankl was probably fundamentally wrong about was his prognosis: "For too long a time—for half a century, in fact—psychiatry tried to interpret the human mind merely as a mechanism, and consequently the therapy of mental disease merely in terms of a technique. I believe this dream has been dreamt out. What now begins to loom on the horizon are not the sketches of a psychologized medicine but rather those of a humanized psychiatry." Unfortunately, the opposite has occurred. Medicine, and at its head psychiatry as the discipline that deals with what constitutes man, his mind and soul, has become mindless and inhumane. I am deeply convinced that there is another way, again following Frankl: "Man is *not* fully conditioned and determined but rather determines himself whether he gives in to conditions or stands up to them. In other words, man is ultimately self-determining. Man does not simply exist but always decides what his existence will be, what he will become in the next moment" [30]. And: not only can it be done differently, it must be done differently. Because otherwise, when we have fulfilled our biological purpose, we will be waiting for our end in a nursing home, cared for by nursing robots, and we will take that for granted.

References

1. New York Times (2013) Angelina Jolie: my medical choice. New York Times, May 14th 2013. https://www.nytimes.com/2013/05/14/opinion/my-medical-choice.html?hp. Accessed on May 11th 2020
2. New York Times (2015) Experts back Angelina Jolie Pitt in choices for cancer prevention. New York Times, March 24th 2015. https://www.nytimes.com/2015/03/25/science/experts-back-angelina-jolie-pitt-in-choices-for-cancer-prevention.html. Accessed on May 11th 2020
3. New York Times (2014) There's cancer in my future. How am i supposed to feel? New York Times, October 19th 2014. https://parenting.blogs.nytimes.com/2014/10/19/theres-cancer-in-my-future-how-am-i-supposed-to-feel/. Accessed on May 11th 2020
4. New York Times (2013) Jolie's disclosure of preventive mastectomy highlights dilemma. New York Times, May 14th 2013. https://www.nytimes.com/2013/05/15/health/angelina-jolies-disclosure-highlights-a-breast-cancer-dilemma.html. Accessed on May 11th 2020
5. Handyside AH, Lesko JG, Tarín JJ et al (1992) Birth of a normal girl after in vitro fertilization and preimplantation diagnostic testing for cystic fibrosis. N Engl J Med 327:905–909

6. Bu G (2009) Apolipoprotein E and its receptors in Alzheimer's disease: pathways, pathogenesis and therapy. Nat Rev Neurosci 10:333–344

7. Corder EH, Saunders AM, Strittmatter WJ et al (1993) Gene dose of apolipoprotein E type 4 allele and the risk of Alzheimer's disease in late onset families. Science 261:921–923

8. Corder EH, Saunders AM, Risch NJ et al (1994) Protective effect of apolipoprotein E type 2 allele for late onset Alzheimer disease. Nat Genet 7:180–184

9. Ripke S et al (2014) Schizophrenia working group of the psychiatric genomics consortium biological insights from 108 schizophrenia-associated genetic loci. Nature 511:421–427

10. Kendler KS (2005) "A gene for…": the nature of gene action in psychiatric disorders. Am J Psychiatry 162:1243–1252

11. Vassos E, Pedersen CB, Murray RM et al (2012) Meta-analysis of the association of urbanicity with schizophrenia. Schizophr Bull 38:1118–1123

12. Jongsma HE, Jones PB (2018) Weaving causal explanations of schizophrenia in urban areas: the role of gene-environment selection. JAMA Psychiatry 75:878–880

13. Jongsma HE, Gayer-Anderson C, Lasalvia A et al (2018) European network of national schizophrenia networks studying gene-environment interactions work package 2 (EU-GEI WP2) group. Treated incidence of psychotic disorders in the multinational EU-GEI study. JAMA Psychiatry 75:36–46

14. Engemann K, Pedersen CB, Agerbo E et al (2020) Association between childhood green space, genetic liability, and the incidence of schizophrenia. Schizophr Bull 46:1629–1637

15. Walters RK, Polimanti R, Johnson EC et al (2018) Transcestral GWAS of alcohol dependence reveals common genetic underpinnings with psychiatric disorders. Nat Neurosci 21:1656–1669

16. Nöthen MM, Degenhardt F, Forstner AJ (2019) Durchbrüche im Verständnis der molekularen Ursachen psychiatrischer Störungen. Nervenarzt 90:99–106

17. McGowan PO, Sasaki A, D'Alessio AC et al (2009) Epigenetic regulation of the glucocorticoid receptor in human brain associates with childhood abuse. Nat Neurosci 12:342–348

18. O'Donnell KJ, Chen L, MacIsaac JL et al (2018) DNA methylome variation in a perinatal nurse-visitation program that reduces child maltreatment: a 27-year follow-up. Transl Psychiatry 8:15

19. Binder EB (2019) Umwelt und Epigenetik. Nervenarzt 90:107–113

20. Turnwald BP, Goyer JP, Boles DZ et al (2019) Learning one's genetic risk changes physiology independent of actual genetic risk. Nat Hum Behav 3:48–56

21. Regalado A (2017) Was the year consumer DNA testing blew up. MIT technology review, February 2nd 2018. https://www.technologyreview.com/s/610233/2017-was-the-year-consumer-dna-testing-blew-up/. Accessed on February 11th, 2020

22. Goodarzi MO (2018) Genetics of obesity: what genetic association studies have taught us about the biology of obesity and its complications. Lancet Diabetes Endocrinol 6:223–236
23. Bessesen DH, Van Gaal LF (2018) Progress and challenges in anti-obesity pharmacotherapy. Lancet Diabetes Endocrinol 6:237–248
24. Deussing JM, Arzt E (2018) P2X7 receptor: a potential therapeutic target for depression? Trends Mol Med 24:736–747
25. Langer EJ (2009) Counterclockwise. A proven way to think yourself younger and healthier. Hodder & Stoughton, London
26. New York Times (2014) What if age is nothing but a mindset? New York Times, October 22nd 2014. https://www.nytimes.com/2014/10/26/magazine/what-if-age-is-nothing-but-a-mind-set.html. Accessed on May 11th 2020
27. World Health Organization (2014) Verfassung der Weltgesundheitsorganisation. WHO. https://www.admin.ch/opc/de/classified-compilation/19460131/201405 080000/0.810.1.pdf. Accessed on May 11th 2020
28. Insel T (2017) Star Neuroscientist Tom Insel Leaves the Google-Spawned Verily for … a Startup? Wired Magazine, November 5th 2017 https://www.wired.com/2017/05/star-neuroscientist-tom-insel-leaves-google-spawned-verily-startup/. Accessed on May 11th 2020
29. Campbell DT (1974) Downward causation in hierarchically organised biological systems. In: Ayala FJ, Dobzhansky T (eds) Studies in the philosophy of biology: reduction and related problems. Macmillan, London, pp 179–186
30. Frankl V (1962) Man's search for meaning. Beacon, Boston

Part III

How Do We Want to Live in the Future? A Counter-Draft to Harari's "Divine Human Being"

We have seen in Chap. 2 that the Israeli historian Harari stands on the point of view that the health and well-being of man of the future will be achieved by interventions in the brain and no longer by improvements in his living conditions. That, he says, is yesterday's prescription. He writes: "Forget economic growth, social reform, and political revolutions—to raise global happiness levels, we need to manipulate human biochemistry." I have argued at length in Chap. 3 that it is naive to believe that we can eradicate mental suffering by better medicines. Aldous Huxley already recognized almost 100 years ago that such attempts must lead to dystopia. Hundreds of millions of people all over the world try every day to reduce their sense of suffering and increase their sense of happiness with substances—alcohol, cocaine, heroin and many others. But this only succeeds in the short term; the end result is usually greater suffering. In this chapter, I will show that there are numerous approaches to (further) improving the world we live in so that depression, anxiety, and addiction become less frequent and ultimately more manageable. To want to abolish mental suffering, however, means to fundamentally question the existence of human beings as they are and, in final consequence, to want to create machine beings. In Chap. 6 we saw that it is basically possible for each individual to take measures for himself to maintain and increase his physical and, above all, his mental health and well-being. But that is not nearly enough. What kind of world would it be in which everyone desperately tries to keep themselves healthy through healthy eating, exercise and meditation techniques, but social conditions steadily deteriorate? That would be as dystopian a vision as the one Harari paints. Only in a world that aims to increase the common good can health and well-being flourish for individuals.

It is our living environment, what surrounds us on a daily basis, how we live, how we work, with whom and how we socialize, that determines quite significantly whether and how satisfied, perhaps happy, we are with our lives. Manipulating the individual brain to increase happiness is doomed to failure, Harari certainly grotesquely misjudged in his utopia of the divine human. How we see the place of ourselves as humans in this world, that is, our fundamental worldview, also influences how we design our health care system. If we see ourselves only as deterministically functioning biomachines, we make ourselves pawns in the concert of medical and IT conglomerates. There are numerous influencing factors of our social environment that significantly determine our physical and especially our mental health—and health is again not understood simply as the absence of disease. We decide whether to intervene in our biochemistry or to maintain and increase our future well-being by shaping our living environment—the design of workplaces, cities, but above all our education system. In this world, people actively shape their own future, creating the framework conditions for their physical and mental health. We really do have a choice!

8

How We Live and Reside

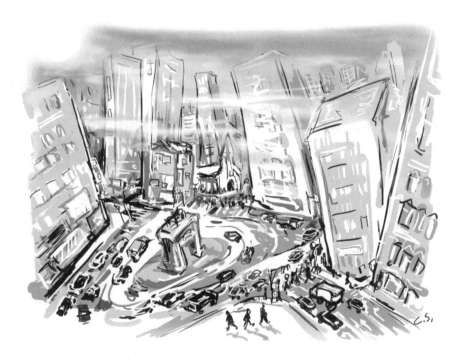

Abstract More and more people are living in cities, and by 2050 almost 70% of the world's population will live there. What means an increase in quality of life for many people who move to cities also poses a challenge. People who grow up in large cities have a higher risk of developing a mental health disorder, and living in cities is associated with increased psychosocial stress. City

G. Gründer, *How Do We Want to Live?*, https://doi.org/10.1007/978-3-662-64225-2_8

dwellers are more likely to develop most mental illnesses. A green environment, in turn, reduces these risks and is associated with better cognitive performance. Planners of the cities of the future, especially in the exploding megacities of Asia and Africa, must take these observations into account if we are not to deal with an ever-increasing burden of disease from mental illness.

According to United Nations figures, only 30% of the world's population lived in cities in 1950; by 2018, this figure had already reached 55% [1]. By 2050, it is expected to rise to 68%. Then, 2.5 billion more people than today could live in cities. 90% of this huge increase in urban population will be in cities in Asia and Africa, a third of which will be in just three countries. In 2050, 400 million *more* people than today will live in cities in India, 250 million in China and almost 200 million in Nigeria. Although Asia today is still much more rural than America or Europe, it already has 54% of the urban population (only 13% in Europe). By contrast, the number of people living in rural areas has increased only slowly since 1950, reaching 3.4 billion in 2018. This number is expected to peak in a few years and then decline to 3.1 billion by 2050. The developments outlined here will therefore hit countries with predominantly low to middle incomes the hardest, presenting them with particular challenges [1].

Today, one in eight people already lives in a megacity with a population of more than ten million. The city with the highest population in 2018 was Tokyo with 37 million, followed by New Delhi with 29 million, Shanghai with 26 million, and Mexico City and Sao Paulo with 22 million each. The next four largest cities, Cairo, Mumbai, Beijing, and Dhaka, each with nearly 20 million residents, are all in Africa and Asia. And while megacities on these continents will continue to grow seemingly inexorably over the next few decades, UN projections predict that Tokyo's population will shrink, with New Delhi expected to replace Tokyo as the most populous city by 2028.

In Germany, as in most countries with higher to high incomes in Europe or North America, development has been far less dynamic than in Asia or Africa, and this will remain the case until 2050. In 1950, 68% of the population in Germany already lived in cities, in 2018 this share had risen to 77%, and in 2050 it will be about 85%. The total population will then have shrunk slightly and will again be below 80 million. There will also continue to be no megacities. In 2018, there were only four megacities in Germany (Berlin, Hamburg, Munich and Cologne), and that will not have changed—at least according to UN estimates—in 2050. And the number of cities with a population between 500,000 and one million—in 2018, there were eleven—will not change either. Well over half of Germany's population will still live in cities in 2050, but they will have fewer than 300,000 inhabitants. This means that the problems associated with urbanization are likely to be far less severe in Germany than in the megacities of Asia and Africa. It is to be feared that there the rapid growth of cities, if the development of socio-economic conditions does not keep pace, will pose particular challenges to human adaptability.

What impact will the increasing urbanisation of our planet have on people's health—especially their mental health? Will the advantages of urban living—e.g. better access to the health and education system, a larger and more differentiated labour market—outweigh the disadvantages? The Berlin psychiatrist Mazda Adli has proposed the term "neurourbanism" for the interdisciplinary collaboration of architecture, urban planning and neuroscience. In his book "Stress and the City" he discusses a variety of findings on the relationship between urbanization and psychological well-being [2]. He describes the aim of neurourban studies as "research into the relationship between social constellations within the city, urban conditions and psychological well-being" [3].

In Chap. 7 I already pointed out that the risk of developing schizophrenia is higher in cities than in rural areas, and it is apparently particularly high in the megacities of the North, e.g. in Paris or London. The relationship between population density and schizophrenia risk is apparently linear: a meta-analysis by British scientists found that the risk in cities with the highest degree of urbanisation is even 2.37-fold higher—i.e. far more than twice as high—than in the most rural regions [4]. There is a clear dose-response relationship. The living environment in the first 15 years of life is of crucial importance: Those who spent this lifetime entirely in an environment with the highest degree of urbanization even have an almost threefold increased risk of schizophrenia, while people who spent their childhood in a rural environment have a reduced risk compared to the average [5]. The renowned Dutch schizophrenia researcher Jim van Os estimates that 30% of the risk of developing schizophrenia is due to the urban environment [6]. Also, in Chap. 7, I had already referred to a large population study from Denmark that concluded that people who spent their childhood in very rural areas have only half the risk of developing schizophrenia as people who grew up in large urban centers without greenery. The effect of childhood living environment was larger than the effect of their polygenetic risk score [7].

However, schizophrenia is not the only mental illness that is more common in people who grew up in (very large) cities. Depression and anxiety disorders, which are particularly common, also occur more often in people who spent their childhood and adolescence in cities. A Dutch team of researchers, in an analysis of all studies that examined the risks of mental illness in urban versus rural populations between 1985 and 2010, found about a 40% increased risk in people who lived in the city. The increase in the risk of affective disorders, which are primarily depressions, was also in this order of magnitude. Addictive disorders, for example alcohol dependence, were excluded from this, as there were no differences in frequency between urban and rural areas [8].

Two studies are available for Germany. In a representative population sample of 4181 persons aged between 18 and 65 years, the frequency of mental illnesses was examined over a 12-month period as a function of the degree of urbanization [9]. The degree of urbanization was divided into five levels, depending on the place of residence. Places with less than 5000 inhabitants were classified as very rural. At the other end ("extremely urban") were the city centers of cities with more than half a million inhabitants, while the suburbs of these metropolitan areas were considered "very urban", as were cities of less than 500,000 inhabitants. Almost all psychiatric disorders were more common among people living in urban environments. Only for substance dependencies and psychoses was such a relationship not found. The fact that psychoses were not more common in urban populations than in rural ones in this study, contrary to what is shown above, is most likely due to methodological reasons (in a sample of only just over 4000 people, psychoses are probably too rare in a 12-month period to find differences). Female sex, low social status and being unmarried were also associated with more psychiatric illness. Being married or living with a partner is also considered a protective factor against psychiatric illness, as is higher social or socioeconomic status . As the degree of urbanization increased, so did the risk of being affected by more than one psychiatric disorder, and the influence of urbanization was evident in all age groups, in both sexes, and in both married and single people [9]. The authors attribute their study results to more stress in urban environmental situations (lack of social cohesion, reduced living space, overstimulation, lower quality housing, more crime). However, they also do not rule out the possibility that 'social drift' may be a contributing factor. As discussed in Chap. 7, the "social drift" hypothesis refers to the selective migration of people with psychiatric disorders to urban settings. However, Andreas Meyer-Lindenberg, director of the Mannheim Central Institute of Mental Health, rules out such social drift as the sole explanation for the greater incidence of mental illness in cities: "Cities are indeed a causal factor for mental disorders, we know that from epidemiological studies. Alternative explanations such as the drift hypothesis, according to which cities attract more psychologically susceptible people, are simply not compatible with the data available. So cities are actually not particularly good for the psyche, which is surprising because they otherwise have quite a lot of positive effects on health." [10]. Meyer-Lindenberg has been studying the impact of the residential environment on mental health for many years. He attributes the higher risk of illness to the higher social stress in the city. I will come back to this in detail below.

The second study that collected figures on the relationship between urbanization and the risk of mental illness in Germany was a comparison of six European countries (Belgium, Germany, France, Italy, the Netherlands, Spain) on this question [11]. In this study, only a very simple distinction was made between rural and urban environments (smaller or larger than 10,000 inhabitants). More than 20,000 people were interviewed regarding the presence of a psychiatric illness in the past twelve months. In this study, too, more psychiatric illnesses were found overall in people who lived in an urban environment. This was especially true for depression, less pronounced for anxiety disorders and not at all for alcohol dependence. However, the differences between urban and rural areas were significant only in Germany and France, and in Belgium psychiatric disorders were even significantly more frequent among the rural population. Interestingly, in Germany and France, significantly fewer married and more divorced people were found in the urban population, and at least for Germany, the authors of the study suggest that the increase in risk among the urban population may be related to their marital status [11]. A significant weakness of the study is certainly that the influence of truly metropolitan life—i.e. in cities with more than at least 100,000 or even 500,000 inhabitants—was not examined here. In addition, the countries studied show considerable differences in the degree of urbanization and population density.

People living in an urban environment are exposed to a variety of stressors. These include physical (e.g. noise), social (high density of people) and emotional (confrontation with aggression and violence) stressors. How these factors associated with urban life cause people to develop depression, anxiety disorders, or even psychosis is only broadly understood. The group led by the Mannheim psychiatrist Meyer-Lindenberg examined healthy people from rural regions, from towns with more than 10,000 inhabitants and from cities with more than 100,000 inhabitants using functional magnetic resonance imaging [12]. In the tomograph, the subjects were subjected to a stress test, i.e. they had to solve arithmetic problems under time pressure while receiving negative feedback on their performance from the study leader. This not only increased their pulse, blood pressure and salivary concentrations of the stress hormone cortisol, but also led to the activation of brain regions that play a central role in the regulation of stress and emotions. Two findings were particularly interesting: the degree of urbanization of the living environment in which the subjects *currently* lived correlated significantly with the stress-induced activation of the so-called amygdala, a brain region that is known to be particularly strongly activated by stress or intense emotions. That is, subjects who lived in the largest cities showed the strongest activation of their amygdala under stress. It has also been known for some years that the amygdala is particularly sensitive to stress in depression, and that this sensitivity is reduced by many antidepressants. The second important finding was that the degree of urbanization of the residential environment in which the subjects had grown up, that is, had spent childhood and adolescence up to the age of 15, correlated with the stress-induced activation of the so-called anterior cingulate cortex (abbreviated ACC). The ACC has an important function in impulse and emotion control, and it is functionally closely related to the amygdala. Subjects who had spent their entire first 15 years of life growing up in the big city showed the strongest activation of their ACC under stress in MRI, and the functional linkage of their ACC to the amygdala was weakest [12]. So it seems undeniable that stress associated with urban living leaves its mark on our brains.

Social stress is one of the stressors with the greatest impact on our health. Both very high social density and social isolation can be experienced as stress. The effects can be particularly impressive when social isolation is experienced in particularly socially dense environments, for example as a migrant in a city with over a million inhabitants. The situation of migrants is therefore a particularly well-studied example of how social isolation increases susceptibility to psychiatric illness. Migrants are significantly more likely to develop schizophrenia than the normal population, and the risk of developing the disease appears to be even higher in the second generation of migrants than in the first [13]. This is particularly true for people whose migrant status is visible, for example, people who have migrated to London from the Caribbean or West Africa, or to The Hague from Morocco. We also know that the risk of disease is particularly elevated when the so-called "ethnic density" is low, that is, when the group to which the migrant belongs is small relative to the population in which he or she moves. These relationships have been shown very consistently by Dutch researchers for The Hague and British researchers for London [14, 15]. In doing so, they ultimately confirmed old findings from 1930s Chicago that African Americans were particularly likely to develop schizophrenia if they lived in neighborhoods with predominantly white populations [16]. These observations suggest that social exclusion and discrimination play an important role in the development of schizophrenia. Higher ethnic density might protect against the consequences of social stress experienced by migrants by facilitating identification with one's ethnic group and reducing exposure to social exclusion by the native population [15].

Social stress, in turn, also has a significant impact on our physical health. I have already indicated in the introductory chapter how closely the experience of stress and physical health are connected. Social stress, however, is possibly the strongest stressor we know. This has been shown in all kinds of animals, including non-human primates, i.e. monkeys. Even mice kept in excessive numbers in small cages become obese without gaining weight, i.e. they increase their fat depots [17].

In primates exposed to chronic social stress, the deposition of so-called "visceral" fat is promoted, which in turn increases the risk of cardiovascular disease [18]. American primate researchers summarized the available evidence to suggest that in humans, social stress and socioeconomic status are inversely related. The growing socioeconomic inequality in many parts of the world thus also leads to an ever-increasing inequality in health [19]. Even the course of cancer is influenced by the social environment, and apparently across all animal species. It influences tumor growth even in fruit flies to an impressive degree. French scientists showed that tumours of the intestinal tract grew most slowly in those flies that were kept with other flies that also carried such a tumour. Tumours grew significantly faster in flies kept in isolation, but fastest in insects kept with tumour-free flies [20]. Similar correlations were found in higher animals. Rats are usually extraordinarily sociable animals. Keeping them in isolation for life has serious consequences. Female rats with a high genetic risk of developing mammary tumors develop more malignant and significantly larger tumors when kept in isolation, and these tumors also spread more frequently than in animals kept in groups appropriate to the species [21]. And in humans, there is also much evidence that chronic stress, depression and social isolation can accelerate tumor growth [22]. However, it is apparently less clear whether chronic stress also increases the risk of developing cancer.

However, there is widespread agreement that a solution to the problem cannot be a "back to the countryside". Such a move would not only entail enormous urban sprawl in rural areas, with many resulting disadvantages. Urban living is also associated with better educational opportunities, better health care, more social stimulation, social participation, and personal development opportunities, and cities form the cultural, social, and political centers of all nations on earth [2, 3, 23]. Nevertheless, on closer inspection, some of the aforementioned advantages of the urban environment turn out to be advantages mainly for those who know how to use the privileges of the city anyway. Would it not be considerably better not to fall ill in the first place than to have to make use of the incomparably denser network of psychotherapists in the city? And the possibilities of "social stimulation and social participation" [3] are particularly well used by those who are socially well connected and socially privileged. It is precisely in the cities that the army of the socially isolated, the isolated and the elderly is growing, and it is precisely these who are particularly at risk. The challenges arising here are enormous, and this is particularly true in the countries of Asia and Africa, whose populations are moving from the countryside to the city to a much greater extent than those in Europe or America, and whose social and health systems appear to be totally inadequately prepared for the changes that are to be expected.

Neurourban studies has identified three broad themes that it intends to address in order to meet the future challenges outlined [3]:

1. Interaction between humans and the urban environment: How does the architecture we are surrounded by influence our psychological well-being? What influence does our urban living space have on our mental health? How does urban planning affect people's ability to actively shape their own living space?
2. Characteristics of urban stress: Which stressors of urban life have negative effects on people's health, which stressors possibly have a stimulating effect and can thus be assessed positively? Which population groups are particularly at risk from urban stress?
3. Socialization, prevention and therapy: What are the particular factors of urban life that make the first 15 years of life particularly significant for later stress sensitivity? How can planning of the built and social urban environment reduce the risk of diseases that are clustered in people living in large cities? What concepts must local policy develop in order to have answers to the challenges of the future?

In order to be able to answer these questions appropriately, Adli and colleagues call for "methodical cooperation between urban planners, architects, sociologists, psychologists and psychiatrists" [3]. There are already a number of findings that should be immediately implemented in planning. For example, the positive health effects of green surroundings must be considered proven, and the studies on this subject are constantly increasing in number [24]. People who live in an environment with green spaces move more and have closer social contacts. Vegetation in the city reduces stress, compensates—at least in part—for air pollution, noise and heat. In addition, there is evidence that the absence of green space is associated with more overweight and obesity, and the children of pregnant women who spend time in green spaces during pregnancy have higher birth weights. Recent data from China also show that living in a greener environment is associated with lower mortality. A Chinese-American research team studied a group of nearly 24,000 very old Chinese (mean age at start of observation 93 years) over a 14-year period and related their mortality rate to the green area of their residence, which they measured using satellite imagery [25]. Individuals living in the "greenest" regions had up to 30% reduced mortality compared to those living in the least green regions.

Spanish scientists studied more than 2500 schoolchildren aged between 7 and 10 years in Barcelona over the course of 12 months by measuring the children's cognitive performance every three months using a computerized test [26]. The researchers measured the extent to which the children were exposed to green spaces at home, at school and on their way to school using high-resolution (5 m × 5 m) satellite images. Children who had more contact with green spaces showed significantly greater increases in working memory performance and greater decreases in inattention over the observation period than children with less exposure to green spaces. However, part of the effect could be explained by differences in air pollution in the respective areas [26]. A study from California even suggests that the frequency of autistic disorders in children may be influenced by the extent of their exposure to green spaces [27].

Similar to Adli from Berlin, Meyer-Lindenberg, the psychiatrist from Mannheim mentioned above, draws clear conclusions from his empirical research. He too calls for close cooperation between urban planners and psychiatrists. In addition to more green spaces in cities, he says, more space is needed for stress-free social interaction: "Places for social interaction are important. There are areas in the city where more social interaction takes place than in others. And there are places that modulate well-being more through social interactions than others. In general, we feel better when we interact with others. But even that varies greatly from individual to individual. The intriguing question is: How do I improve social interactions when I know that in the city the packing density is higher but the social network is smaller than in the countryside?" [10].

References

1. United Nations, Department of Economic and Social Affairs, Population Division. 2018 Revision of World Urbanization Prospects. UN. https://www.un.org/development/desa/publications/2018-revision-of-world-urbanization-prospects.html. Accessed on May 12th, 2020

2. Adli M (2017) Stress and the city. C. Bertelsmann, München
3. Adli M, Berger M, Brakemeier EL et al (2016) Neurourbanistik – ein methodischer Schulterschluss zwischen Stadtplanung und Neurowissenschaften. Die Psychiatrie 13:70–78
4. Vassos E, Pedersen CB, Murray RM et al (2012) Meta-analysis of the association of urbanicity with schizophrenia. Schizophr Bull 38:1118–1123
5. Pedersen CB, Mortensen PB (2001) Evidence of a dose-response relationship between urbanicity during upbringing and schizophrenia risk. Arch Gen Psychiatry 58:1039–1046
6. van Os J (2004) Does the urban environment cause psychosis? Br J Psychiatry 184:287–288
7. Engemann K, Pedersen CB, Agerbo E et al (2020) Association between childhood green space, genetic liability, and the incidence of schizophrenia. Schizophr Bull 46:1629–1637
8. Peen J, Schoevers RA, Beekman AT, Dekker J (2010) The current status of urban-rural differences in psychiatric disorders. Acta Psychiatr Scand 121:84–93
9. Dekker J, Peen J, Koelen J et al (2008) Psychiatric disorders and urbanization in Germany. BMC Public Health 8:17
10. Ärzte-Zeitung (2020) Städte sind nicht gut für die Psyche. Ärzte-Zeitung, 7. Februar
11. Kovess-Masféty V, Alonso J, de Graaf R, Demyttenaere K (2005) A European approach to rural-urban differences in mental health: the ESEMeD 2000 comparative study. Can J Psychiatr 50:926–936
12. Lederbogen F, Kirsch P, Haddad L et al (2011) City living and urban upbringing affect neural social stress processing in humans. Nature 474:498–501
13. Cantor-Graae E, Selten JP (2005) Schizophrenia and migration: a meta-analysis and review. Am J Psychiatry 162:12–24
14. Boydell J, van Os J, McKenzie K et al (2001) Incidence of schizophrenia in ethnic minorities in London: ecological study into interactions with environment. BMJ 323:1336–1338
15. Veling W, Susser E, van Os J et al (2008) Ethnic density of neighborhoods and incidence of psychotic disorders among immigrants. Am J Psychiatry 165:66–73
16. Faris R, Dunham HW (1939) Mental disorders in urban areas. University of Chicago Press, Chicago
17. Lin EJ, Sun M, Choi EY et al (2015) Social overcrowding as a chronic stress model that increases adiposity in mice. Psychoneuroendocrinology 51:318–330
18. Shively CA, Register TC, Clarkson TB (2009) Social stress, visceral obesity, and coronary artery atherosclerosis: product of a primate adaptation. Am J Primatol 71:742–751
19. Shively CA, Day SM (2014) Social inequalities in health in nonhuman primates. Neurobiol Stress 1:156–163
20. Dawson EH, Bailly TPM, Dos Santos J et al (2018) Social environment mediates cancer progression in Drosophila. Nat Commun 9:3574

21. Hermes GL, Delgado B, Tretiakova M et al (2009) Social isolation dysregulates endocrine and behavioral stress while increasing malignant burden of spontaneous mammary tumors. Proc Natl Acad Sci USA 106:22393–22398
22. Moreno-Smith M, Lutgendorf SK, Sood AK (2010) Impact of stress on cancer metastasis. Future Oncol 6:1863–1881
23. Meyer WB (2013) The environmental advantages of cities: countering commonsense antiurbanism. MIT Press, Cambridge
24. Fong KC, Hart JE, James P (2018) A review of epidemiologic studies on greenness and health: updated literature through 2017. Curr Environ Health Rep 5:77–87
25. Ji JS, Zhu A, Bai C et al (2019) Residential greenness and mortality in oldest-old women and men in China: a longitudinal cohort study. Lancet Planet Health 3:e17–e25
26. Dadvand P, Nieuwenhuijsen MJ, Esnaola M et al (2015) Green spaces and cognitive development in primary schoolchildren. Proc Natl Acad Sci USA 112:7937–7942
27. Wu J, Jackson L (2017) Inverse relationship between urban green space and childhood autism in California elementary school districts. Environ Int 107:140–146

9

How We Work

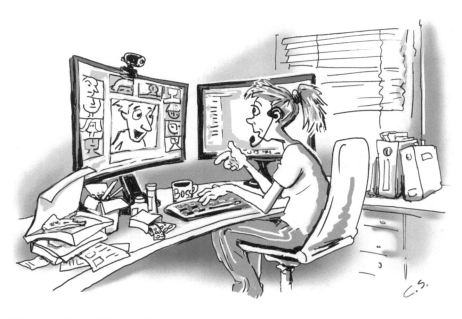

Abstract Probably nothing has changed our daily lives more in the last 30 years than the way we work. The internet and email, as ubiquitous signs of technologization and globalization, have accelerated our working lives in a way that only the over-50s can appreciate. The impact of this acceleration on our mental health can hardly be overestimated. It is above all those people who are well connected and live from and with digitalisation who suffer particularly from the stress associated with it. Technologization and globalization

G. Gründer, *How Do We Want to Live?*, https://doi.org/10.1007/978-3-662-64225-2_9

also lead to increasing isolation. Networking and the worldwide mobility of millions of well-educated young people from economically emerging countries threaten prosperity and social peace in the countries of the industrialized world. Together, these accelerating global trends pose significant challenges to our mental health that we will need to address proactively.

How we work has changed dramatically over the last 30 years, and all the evidence suggests that the pace of change is likely to accelerate in the future. This has implications for our mental (and, by all accounts in this book, consequently our physical) health that cannot be overestimated. We will also have to meet the challenges of these dramatically changing work environments in order to stay healthy. In her book "The Shift—the future of work is already here", British management professor Lynda Gratton describes five forces that will determine the future of our working world [1]. Gratton is probably one of the most knowledgeable academics when it comes to the topic of the future of work. For many years, she has led an international group of international companies and academics, the Future of Work Consortium, which has not only analyzed the problem but also presented approaches to possible solutions. Accordingly, these five defining forces are:

- Technology
- Globalization
- Demography and life expectancy
- Society
- Energy resources

For me personally—from my point of view as a psychiatrist—the most important reason for the enormous changes in the world of work, which I already briefly discussed in Chap. 2, is the technologization of our world, especially digitalization. Closely linked to this is the trend towards globalization. What politicians like to praise in soapbox speeches as the solution to all problems—and we know this quite well by now—also poses a threat to our mental health. When I started my first job at a psychiatric university hospital in 1989 as a young resident (at that time it was just called "doctor in internship"; there were enough doctors, which is why they could be paid like interns; there was even talk of a "doctor glut"), there was neither email nor internet, not to mention "social media". Mail was delivered twice a day at the hospital, so you had a post box at the gate where you picked up your mail twice a day. Otherwise, one had time to concentrate on one's tasks in patient care and research. News was available in the morning in the printed newspaper or in the evening on television. Nevertheless, at least in retrospect, one did not feel any less informed than today. If you wanted to send documents particularly quickly, you had to fax them. There was a single, centrally located fax machine in the clinic. If you wanted to do a literature search for your scientific paper, you had to go to the library and laboriously search through microfiche catalogs. People who are now younger than 40 or possibly even 50 will no longer even know what that is. Then, when you had completed a publication manuscript after your scientific work was done, you sent it to a scientific journal—as a printed versatile document in the mail! If the journal was an American one, it could easily take a week for your work to reach the recipient. This was then sent—again by post, of course—to reviewers spread around the world. So you knew you had to be patient for a few months until you got word from the journal whether your work was being considered for publication. Mobile phones didn't exist yet either, at least not for everyone. I got my first cell phone in 1996, and back then you were considered—no joke—a snobby poser if you showed up on the street with one. So when you went home, the best you could be reached for was to leave your landline number at the clinic (or wherever else it was needed) for any emergency. This was even more true for holidays: You were simply away and unavailable to anyone, and you didn't have to feel guilty about it, because no one seriously expected you to call your boss every day from an Italian phone booth and ask if there was anything important to do. Even if you were professionally ambitious, life was relatively quiet because of the lack of fast communication channels. Nor did one constantly compare one's successes (or failures) with those of colleagues elsewhere, because the possibilities for doing so were simply not available. Scientific output, which in science then as now is measured by the number of publications of the highest possible rank, was much lower, partly because all processes were slower, but also because the world was much less networked.

I am not telling you anything new when I say that the world has accelerated dramatically in just one or two decades. Rarely, however, do people realize the changes that this acceleration has brought to their own lives. The most obvious sign is the constant bombardment of information to which we are exposed. Today I receive not three, five or ten letters, but 50 to 100 emails a day. Some are just part of bulk emails to a large group of recipients, but most require an individual response. The speed of this information channel also means that a prompt response is expected. Unlike 30 or even 25 years ago, when the possibilities simply didn't exist, today academics and executives in particular continue to communicate, read and write even after "closing time", often on weekends, even when the email bombardment dies down. And often they don't stop even when they're on vacation. This leads to the fact that, as I explained in Chap. 2, it is precisely those people who are well digitally networked who feel particularly stressed. Technology and digitalization have thus led to an enormous fragmentation of our working lives. So while 30 years ago people sometimes sat undisturbed for several hours on a task, today's working day of people in the information and service sector consists of fragments of three (!) minutes. Today, the working day does not begin at the workplace and end when I leave it, as was the case for me in 1990; it usually begins shortly after getting up, reading the emails and messages received during the night, and for many it ends in the evening on the sofa at home, or, not uncommonly, even in bed, writing the last messages. This fragmentation of our working days has led to a dramatic reduction in our attention span and concentration. Time for reflection, observation, even mind games and building castles in the air, is hardly available today, time that is necessary for creativity to flourish. The people of Generation Y, i.e. those born between 1980 and 1995, and even less so Generation Z, born after that, don't know any different. Lynda Gratton uses the image of the frog being boiled for the changes that occurred in our working lives between 1990 and 2000. If you throw a frog into a container of boiling water, it immediately jumps out of the container with a horrified jump. If, on the other hand, you put the frog into a vessel of cold water and heat it very slowly, it will be boiled alive [1]. This is how a person from the baby boomer generation feels, who still got to know a completely different pace at work and today wonders how one could adapt to this fragmentation without complaint.

Another consequence of technologization, digitalization and globalization is the increasing isolation in which we do our work. We are experiencing this in extreme form at the moment of the politically imposed social distancing necessitated by the rapid spread of the SARS-CoV 2 virus. In the space of two weeks, a significant part of my work has shifted to video conferencing. So has everyone who normally spends their work at desks behind computer screens, and this is a group of the working population that has grown in size over the last 20 years. And with digitalization, it will continue to grow. With the arrival of robots in our lives, even surgeons will be able to do their work at home on a computer in just a few years, controlling a surgical robot from there that will most certainly have a steady hand. More and more of our social relationships, which have determined our working lives throughout the development of mankind, are being transferred to the digital world. Interestingly, this is also being driven by more sustainable environmental policies that will make it increasingly necessary in the future to forgo travel, especially travel across continents, and instead exchange ideas via video conferencing. My first real "virtual conference", enforced by the quite acute global travel ban, took place on March 19, 2020. I was invited to speak in Vienna at a conference on "Homo digitalis," on a couple of the topics I have critically discussed in this book. So I would have spoken in a venerable lecture hall of the University of Vienna in front of a planned audience of 70–80 people, I would have come into contact with them, not only with glances, but with my whole physical presence, one would have really met. So now the conference had been cancelled a few days before the planned date, and I talked to my screen at home, where a few faces could be seen in a few small windows, barely more than postage stamp-sized, and the people behind those faces might listen to me, or they might not. Will this be the future of the scientific meeting? I hope not. People like to refer to meetings where people still actually physically meet as "face-to-face" meetings. But that is a very misleading term. I see a "face" on my screen, but when I actually meet someone, it's much more than two faces exchanging words. It's a complex social interaction, a connection. The current so-called "Corona crisis" made that abundantly clear after just two weeks. People feel lonely, they crave the personal contact in convivial company, even the physical touch. It is completely inconceivable that this kind of human interaction can be shifted to the digital world. Such a development would make us deeply unhappy. However, this aspect of the future of work is not limited to our working world; it encompasses our entire social interaction. I will therefore return to it in the next chapter ("How we live together"). But what I would like to emphasize again at this point: Who would really believe that I could adapt man, really considered as an individual, to these new social structures, as the vision of "Homo deus" would have us believe? Unhappiness here arises not in the individual, but from the (lack of!) interaction of individuals. The social structure is the problem, not the brain chemistry of the individual.

A second major reason for the change in our working lives is actually a good one: we are getting older and older. We already read in Chap. 2 that average life expectancy has risen from 31 years in 1800 to 72 years today, and that there is not a single country in the world today where it is less than 50 years. Over the past 200 years, life expectancy has increased by about two years every decade. And these trends continue. A child born today has a 50% chance of living to 105. For a child born one hundred years ago, that prospect was 1%. If you are 20 years old today, you have a 50% chance of living to 100, and if you are already 60 years old today, you have the same chance of living to 90. Lynda Gratton and her colleague Andrew Scott explain in their book "The 100-year life" [2] that our ever-longer lifespans will present us with very special challenges in the future. This is, of course, also due to the fact that our working world is changing ever faster. It is already becoming increasingly unlikely that we will continue in a job we learned in young adulthood until retirement, and in the future this will be almost impossible. Work biographies as we still know them from our parents (usually our fathers, in fact) will no longer exist. My own father spent practically his entire working life—more than 40 years (!)—with just one employer, in one company, after completing his vocational training. Today, entire branches of industry are disappearing within a few years (e.g. coal mining), while others are undergoing enormous structural change (e.g. the car industry with its move away from the combustion engine towards alternative forms of propulsion). In this rapidly changing world of work, those who are not willing or able to constantly adapt and continue to learn will run the risk of being overtaken and replaced by the mass of young, up-and-coming global workers who have qualified themselves in line with the prevailing requirements. There is also no doubt that we will have to work longer than we do now. It is simply inconceivable that we will continue to retire at age 67 (which is the retirement age in Germany for all those born after 1964, and regardless of age) if we are then to receive benefits from the statutory pension scheme for 20 or more years. When Imperial Chancellor Otto von Bismarck introduced pension insurance in Germany, in 1891, the retirement age was 70; in 1911 it was lowered to 65. At that time, however, almost no one reached that age. The pension insurance system, and with it the retirement age, will have to take account of the development of the age structure everywhere in the world. So it will be inevitable that we will not only have to work longer; we will also have to learn for much longer if we are to cope in rapidly changing working environments.

There are other major problems in the future world of work that are outside the focus of this book. Lynda Gratton has analysed them in her book and also pointed out possible solutions. It is clear that the world of work will change enormously in the next few years. Globalization and technologization will lead to social upheavals in the Western world, the explosive power of which we probably have no idea about yet. By 2020, the populations of China and India will each exceed 1.4 billion people. A growing number of them, many, many millions and growing, are highly educated; they are already competing, in a globalized and digitized world, with the elites of the Western industrialized nations. Whereas until the end of the twentieth century it was still possible to earn a living in a European country or in the USA without any special training, jobs that do not require education or training will increasingly fall victim to automation. In the future, being born in a Western industrialized country will no longer mean somehow making a living. Prosperity and poverty will no longer be distinguishing features of the developed and developing world; they will divide all populations globally. The increasing global competition that each individual will face even in their schooling will increase the stress of workers, and with the stress will increase the fear of failure and of not being able to maintain one's own standard of living, or that of one's parents. The sense of anxiety has increased in American society between 1952 and 1993, and exponentially at that. In 1993, the average American college student suffered more anxiety than 85% of the population in 1952 [3]. This trend continues into the new millennium. California psychologist Jean Twenge attributes this to changes in culture, which has increasingly moved away from intrinsic human goals such as community, meaning in life, and relationships toward extrinsic motives such as materialism and status [4]. No one can really think that countering this increasing existential anxiety with depressant or anxiety-relieving drugs is a successful strategy.

However, the trend towards automation, which will threaten the very existence of the less educated and less trained in particular, has already significantly changed the lives of all working people in the industrialised countries. An enormous amount of free time has been created. What do we do with all this "free time"? The average American watched four hours and 46 min of television in 2018, and people over the age of 65, i.e. those in retirement, spent a staggering 7 h and 24 min in front of the television. This also makes Americans the world champions in this discipline. Younger people have clearly shifted their media consumption to the Internet; people up to 35 years of age watch only 2 h and 17 min of television. The average German watches about an hour less TV than the American, and his or her online time has probably come into line with that of the American. In the next section ("How We Live Together"), I'll revisit this topic in greater detail. Here, however, we will first focus on how and how wisely we use the time we gain. What will we do with our time if in the future machines and robots do the tedious work for us? This is not an entirely far-fetched utopia, and here it is perhaps particularly true that what some will experience as a blessing will become a curse for others. The more educated part of the population will use the time for personal development and creative work. But the people whose work has been rationalized away by computers and robots will spend more and more of their lives in passive media consumption, and that will not make them any happier. Changes in our working world will in many ways—as I have tried to show here—make significant demands on our mental coping abilities.

References

1. Gratton L (2011) The shift. The future of work is already here. Harper Collins, London
2. Gratton L, Scott A (2016) The 100-year life. Bloomsbury, London
3. Twenge JM (2000) The age of anxiety? Birth cohort change in anxiety and neuroticism, 1952–1993. J Pers Soc Psychol 79:1007–1021
4. Twenge JM, Gentile B, DeWall CN et al (2010) Birth cohort increases in psychopathology among young Americans, 1938–2007: a cross-temporal meta-analysis of the MMPI. Clin Psychol Rev 30:145–154

10

How We Live Together

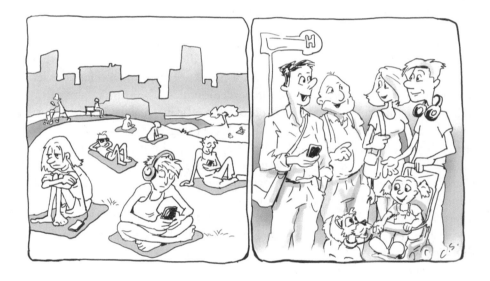

Abstract The industrialized nations of this world are particularly threatened by the modern epidemic of social isolation and loneliness. Loneliness increases our risk of depression and dementia, and it shortens our life expectancy. Loneliness is not a problem of the individual, which can therefore be solved by an individual intervention (e.g. a pharmaceutical), but one of social organization. Causes of the epidemic increase in loneliness include the rapid growth of technology and social media, globalization, and the polarization of societies. Technology and globalization have increased the quality of life

G. Gründer, *How Do We Want to Live?*, https://doi.org/10.1007/978-3-662-64225-2_10

worldwide to a significant degree, but at the same time they have changed social interaction and destroyed traditional social connections. This threat to our mental health must also be addressed.

At various points in this book, I have pointed out that the U.S. society in particular has struggled with rising suicide rates and even dramatically increased death rates from opioid overdoses over the past 20 years. I described how I was also motivated to write this book—among a few other key experiences—by an academic symposium in December 2018 that was supposed to be about "solutions" to the opioid crisis. I reported on where six leading American scientists see their "solution" to the problem: In a better understanding of brain chemistry and pharmacology. Of course, there are other opinions and attitudes about this, and they are finally getting into the top American psychiatric journals. One of America's leading psychiatrists recently wrote: "Since ancient times, millions of people have died from epidemics of plague, influenza, cholera, and other infections caused by bacteria, viruses, or other microorganisms. Major advances in medicine have largely eliminated these mass killers with vaccines and antibiotics. However, modern societies face a new kind of epidemics—*behavioral* epidemics. The annual rates of mortality from suicides and opioid overdose have been escalating over the past two decades, and today are responsible for ending the life of one American every five and a half minutes" [1]. I am writing these lines in mid-March 2020, when there is a worldwide panic because of the new Covid 19 virus. Across Europe, schools and kindergartens, shops and restaurants, sports stadiums and museums, even entire countries are being shut down. To date, more than 5000 people have died from infection with the virus, and the numbers are rising daily, leading to a global panic. The "behavioral epidemics" kill insidiously, yet just as efficiently, but they barely reach the consciousness of the general population. Loneliness is a subjective feeling caused by a mismatch between the desired and perceived number and quality of a person's social relationships. Social isolation, in contrast, is an objective measure of the number of people in a person's environment. We had already noted in Chap. 5 that loneliness and social isolation are considered risk factors for the development of dementia. However, it goes much further than that. Loneliness probably shortens our lives at least as much as smoking or obesity. In the US, 162,000 deaths a year are linked to loneliness, which is more victims than lung cancer claims, for example [2]. According to a recent study, three-quarters of the adult population of California feel at least moderately affected by loneliness.

But the problem is not, of course, an American one. The British government addressed the importance of social isolation and loneliness by appointing a Minister for Loneliness (Tracey Crouch) in January 2018. In October 2018, then UK Prime Minister Theresa May published her strategy for tackling the problem. "Loneliness is one of the biggest public health challenges of our time, Theresa May said today as she launched the first cross-Government strategy to tackle it" the UK government wrote on its website on October 15th, 2018 [3]. According to their surveys, 200,000 older-aged Britons would not have had a conversation with a friend or relative in the last month. Up to 20% of all adults in the UK suffered from loneliness most of the time or permanently. Three quarters of all GPs see between one and five patients a day who are affected by loneliness. The UK government's programme is remarkable and far-sighted, encompassing numerous measures [3]. Not only does it envisage that by 2023 all GPs in the UK will be able to prescribe participation in community activities and voluntary services. The importance of loneliness and the value of social relationships are to be taught as early as in primary schools.

The British daily "The Guardian" commented on the announcement of the establishment of a Ministry of Loneliness a few days later in a remarkable article: "Neither is it [loneliness] an end-of-life condition. Rather it is an indiscriminate disease that has become an epidemic. There are some obvious pathogens: the deconstruction of community, the conversion of citizen into consumer, the politics of envy. We are no longer "bowling together" and family life has been unravelling for some time now. Since the 1980s we've been gaining comfort from consumer materialism and convenience in exchange for our identity. The public square has become privatised and we have lived individual, unconnected lives behind locked doors in gated estates, as we gorge on delivered groceries, box sets and now Just Eat takeaways. We have been slowly losing touch with each other and with reality. The latest strain is a digital virus, detectable only to the analogue eye of our pre-electronic generation. It is demolishing real sociability and replacing it with virtual reality. A techie elite has hijacked the narrative, causing a quantum shift in human interaction" [4].

In an article for the same newspaper, British historian Fay Bound Alberti highlighted that the word loneliness did not exist in the English language until 1800. She writes: "People lived in small communities, they tended to believe in God (which meant they were never really alone, even when they were physically isolated), and there was a philosophical concept of the community as a source of common good. There was no need for a language of loneliness" [5]. Of course, there had been loneliness in the sense of isolation, and it had had just as damaging consequences for the individual then as it does today. However, "But the modern, existential angst of feeling alone couldn't exist, because the modern "individual" didn't emerge until the nineteenth century, with industrialisation in the west and the creation of philosophical and political systems focusing on individualism. Scientific medicine separated mind and body, identifying the brain as the organ of both cognition and mind. Pathological emotions were defined as "mental" problems" [5].

What are the causes of the epidemic increase in loneliness? This results from the rapid growth of technology, social media, globalization and polarization of societies [1]. Hans Rosling would state that technology and globalization have increased the quality of life worldwide to a significant degree. However, at the same time, they have also changed social interaction and destroyed traditional social connections. The constant barrage of information permanently upon us, constant accessibility, relationships that are permanent but superficial via "social" media, and fierce, often global, professional competition have led to a steady increase in stress. Already in Chap. 2, you will remember, we made this diagnosis in the "Stress Report" of one of the large German health insurance companies. It is remarkable that especially those people feel particularly stressed who are employed, and here especially the well-educated. This is just as true for Germans as it is for US Americans. In the Global Emotions 2019 Report by the Gallup polling institute, citizens of the USA were one of the most stressed societies on earth [6].

The historian Alberti demands that a health care system that wants to meet challenges such as the loneliness epidemic must finally evolve from a curative to a preventive system [5]. There will never be a pill for the *causes of* loneliness. There may be a pill for the *feeling of loneliness*, for the malaise and sadness that accompany it. People fight the feeling of loneliness more than ever with antidepressants, alcohol, sometimes with much harder drugs, far too often with food. Aldous Huxley has people turning to the drug "soma" in his dystopia, and more recently, in the heyday of reductionist neurocentrism, Yuval Harari is celebrated by millions for prophesying that we are only a small step away from being able to induce "global happiness," absolute happiness for everyone, through perfect medication. What a naive notion!

Many recent authors agree that it is precisely the so-called "social media" that have fundamentally changed our coexistence and our social relationships for the worse, at least when they are used in excess. Even the United Nations' latest World Happiness Report 2019, which I will return to in more detail later in this chapter, addresses this issue in a separate chapter [7]. It is primarily the American psychologist Jean Twenge, who teaches and works in San Diego, who has devoted a great deal of attention to this topic in recent years.

She has also written the relevant chapter in the World Happiness Report 2019, entitled "The sad state of happiness in the United States and the role of digital media". According to the report, happiness has been declining steadily among Americans since 2011, even though they have been doing better and better economically since surviving the global recession in 2009. This trend is particularly striking among young people. I had already shown in Chap. 2 that the frequency of depression and, particularly alarming, of suicides among adolescents has increased significantly since about 2010, especially among girls. Possible explanations are a decrease in social support and an increase in obesity and drug use. For years, however, Twenge has favoured a different explanation: Americans in general, but young people in particular, spend their leisure time very differently today than they used to. She aptly describes the trends taking place here as "the rise of digital media and the fall of everything else" [7]. Over the past decade, the amount of time young people spent on screens (computer games, social media, texting via messenger) has been steadily increasing; in 2017, this time amounted to more than six hours per day for 17 to 18 year olds, with 45% of respondents reporting being online virtually non-stop. At the same rate, time spent in direct, face-to-face social contact decreased. In addition, less time was spent reading books and magazines, and sleep duration also decreased. Several studies indicate that the duration of digital media use correlates negatively with well-being. Girls who use social media for more than five hours are three times more likely to suffer from depression than girls who abstain completely from social media [8]. It is often pointed out that such correlations are correlative and do not prove causality. It could also be, for example, that young girls and women who are depressed tend to spend more time on social media. However, two observations support causality in the other direction (i.e., excessive social media use leads to reduced well-being): Several longitudinal studies in which individuals were followed over time and their social media use was recorded show that intensity of use predicts *subsequent* well-being [9]. In addition, two randomized trials are now available in which subjects were drawn into two experimental groups. In one study, they continued to use Facebook as before, while the other suspended use for just one week. Subjects in the group that had been prescribed "Facebook holidays" reported more well-being and less depression at the end of the week [10]. In the second study, participants in the group that was told to spend less time on social media were told to spend no more than ten minutes per platform and no more than 30 min per day total on all platforms. The other group continued their use unchanged. This study also showed that the subjects who reduced their social media use reported increased well-being and less loneliness over the course of several weeks [11].

These studies suggest that the relationship between depression and social media use is indeed a causal one. Moreover, it is important to note that the increase in the prevalence of depression among adolescents coincides with the explosion of smartphone use. The idea that the increase in adolescent depression has led to increased smartphone purchases sounds outright absurd. However, there are definitely voices that dispute the fundamentally negative impact of social media use on human well-being. Used correctly and in moderation—that is, above all, actively shaping and not passively consuming—social media could even contribute to increasing well-being [12]. In the meantime, social media have become so integrated into our culture that it is no longer simply a matter of reducing the time spent using them. Rather, it is now necessary to understand the mechanisms through which social media unfold their effects on the human psyche. Then interventions can be developed that change the way they are used in order to capitalize on their positive aspects. In this way, one might even be able to develop personalized interventions, tailored to the individual, to capitalize on the positive potential that social media hold [12]. You will recall that this is the modern trend in psychiatry: if only I understand the mechanism by which humans function in as much detail as possible, then I can purposefully intervene in the mechanism to correct potential flaws in the system. In this way, even tools that have a harmful potential for many young people become means with even therapeutic effects.

How important will personal contact be to us in the future? Many companies around the world are working on care robots, which are supposed to take over the care of old people in particular, because they are cheaper and less demanding than human caregivers. The "robot light" are avatars that you can already book in the USA if you feel lonely (or rather: if you have old relatives for whom you don't have enough time). The Californian company Care. Coach, for example, offers a service that provides round-the-clock care for patients with chronic illnesses. Here, people talk to a computer-animated character (a cat or dog) that allows automated, algorithm-driven conversation about everyday topics. Should the "cared for" person express life-threatening thoughts in their "conversation" with the computer, caregivers or family members are automatically alerted. Loneliness, from which the elderly in particular suffer to a considerable degree, is combated by an avatar on a computer screen or tablet. Are these the answers that psychiatry has for the enormous problems that have arisen due to demographic and changes in our social relationships?

One can also argue about whether psychotherapy can be conducted digitally, for example via a video link between patient and therapist, just as well as in a real, face-to-face conversation. This is a controversial discussion, especially in Germany. At a time when people are being forced by their governments to shut themselves off from each other because of a virus pandemic, digitally mediated therapy sessions may be a good, and often the only, way of establishing therapeutic contact with each other. However, I personally believe that even with this kind of communication, important parts of the personal relationship are lost. In the simplest case, psychotherapy only takes place through the exchange of linguistic signals. Here people meet who exchange many different signals with each other, also in a physical relationship (and "physical" should in no way be misunderstood as "sexual" here). Digital therapies reduce the many different communication channels of human interaction to two (speech and video) or, in extreme cases, even to just one channel (speech). This, by the way, is another example of our culture's perception of mind and body as separate. Psychotherapy is understood here as therapy of the mind, which can proceed with complete disregard for the body. It is the mind that is treated, not the person. Scientific research will have to show in the future whether psychotherapies conducted digitally are as effective as therapies in which people meet in person.

However, I have great doubts as to whether a genuine therapeutic relationship can develop with a machine that takes on the role of psychotherapist. But this is also being worked on. Many people working on artificial intelligence (and, interestingly, many psychiatrists) even believe that psychiatry is the medical discipline that will be taken over most quickly by machines. American and Chinese scientists in particular are working on computers or robots that should eventually be able to perform formal psychotherapy themselves. For the moment, they are still referred to as "conversational agents". Once again, however, the interaction between humans and machines is based exclusively on the communication of text, that is, the machine interprets semantics. Human interaction, after all, goes far beyond semantics; relationships depend on context. How do you encode empathy in words? While generations of psychologists, psychotherapists, and psychoanalysts have tried to understand the multi-layered dynamics of interaction between two (and sometimes more) people, today we think of it only as an exchange of communication signals that can be described by computer algorithms. While, as we have seen in many places in this book, scientific evidence shows that social contact probably plays the most significant role in psychological and physical well-being, we are shaping a world along the lines of "homo deus": a world in which machines are supposed to fulfill basic human needs, the needs for contact, proximity, and unity. A remarkable article in the New York Times some time ago, entitled "Human contact is now a luxury good," said: "Life for all but the very rich—the physical experience of living, learning and dying—is increasingly mediated by screens. Screens themselves are not only cheap to make, they make things cheaper. Any place a screen can be placed (classrooms, hospitals, airports, restaurants) can cut costs. And any activity that can take place on a screen becomes cheaper. The texture of life, the tactile experience, becomes smooth glass. The rich don't live that way. The rich have developed a fear of screens. They want their kids to play with blocks, and tech-free private schools are booming. People are more expensive and rich people are willing and able to pay for it. Conspicuous human interaction—living a day without a phone, leaving social networks, not answering emails—has become a status symbol" [13]. How much truth is contained here was recently confirmed by a scientific article in a renowned American journal: "Computer therapists" are particularly helpful in psychiatrically "underserved populations" [14]—read: the poor and uneducated.

In the future, how likely will I be to spend the next 50, 60, 70, or even 80 years together with the person with whom I start a family and have children in my third decade of life [15]? There are many factors that have caused divorce rates to rise around the world in recent decades. Rising life expectancy is likely to play an increasingly important role in the future. While the divorce rate in Germany was only about 10% in 1960, it rose to more than 50% by 2005. Since then it has fallen again to around 33%, meaning that there is one divorce for every three marriages. The figures for the US show similar trends. However, looking at the divorce rate only relates the number of marriages to the number of divorces in a given year. That is, it does not allow a direct conclusion to be drawn about the risk of a marriage being divorced, because that would require tracking all marriages in a defined year over the long run. A falling divorce rate is at least partly faked by the fact that the number of marriages has fallen sharply over the last 15 years. Thinking about how we will live together in the future—especially in a world where we are getting older—may also mean rethinking couple relationships. As recently as the 1800s, as we've heard many times before, the average life expectancy was only 31 years. Decades-long partnerships were simply the absolute exception in that era. The analysis of what our ever-increasing life expectancy means for our partnerships is beyond the focus of this book; it has been done by others [15]. But it must be clear to us that the stability and duration of our couple relationships have crucial importance for our psychological well-being. And our partnerships can also only be influenced to a very limited extent by individual brain chemistry.

References

1. Jeste DV, Lee EE, Cacioppo S (2020) Battling the modern behavioral epidemic of loneliness. Suggestions for research and interventions. JAMA Psychiatry 77:553–554

2. Veazie S, Gilbert JA, Winchell K, Paynter R, Guise J-M (2019) Addressing social isolation to improve the health of older adults: a rapid review. Rockville, MD: AHRQ. https://effectivehealthcare.ahrq.gov/sites/default/files/pdf/rapid-social-isolation-older-adults-final.pdf. Accessed on May 13th 2020

3. GOV.UK (2018) PM [Prime Minister] launches Government's first loneliness strategy. Oktober 15th 2018. https://www.gov.uk/government/news/pm-launches-governments-first-loneliness-strategy. Accessed on May 13th 2020

4. The Guardian (2018) The minister for loneliness will need all the friends she can get. January 23rd 2018. https://www.theguardian.com/society/2018/jan/23/tracey-crouch-minister-loneliness-friends-powerful-vested-interests. Accessed on May 13th 2020

5. The Guardian (2018) Loneliness is a modern illness of the body, not just the mind. November 1st 2018. https://www.theguardian.com/commentisfree/2018/nov/01/loneliness-illness-body-mind-epidemic. Accessed on May 13th 2020

6. Gallup (2019) Global emotions report. https://www.gallup.com/analytics/248909/gallup-2019-global-emotions-report-pdf.aspx. Accessed on May 13th 2020

7. Helliwell JF, Layard R, Sachs JD (2019) World happiness report. (https://s3.amazonaws.com/happiness-report/2019/WHR19.pdf. Accessed on May 13th 2020

8. Kelly Y, Zilanawala A, Booker C, Sacker A (2019) Social media use and adolescent mental health: findings from the UK Millennium Cohort Study. EClin Med. https://www.thelancet.com/journals/eclinm/article/PIIS2589-5370(18)30060-9/fulltext. Accessed on May 13th 2020

9. Shakya HB, Christakis NA (2017) Association of facebook use with compromised well-being: a longitudinal study. Am J Epidemiol 185:203–211

10. Tromholt M (2016) The Facebook experiment: quitting facebook leads to higher levels of well-being. Cyberpsychol Behav Soc Netw 19:661–666

11. Hunt MG, Marx R, Lipson C, Young J (2018) No more FOMO: limiting social media decreases loneliness and depression. J Social Clin Psychol 37:751–768

12. Timpano KR, Beard C (2020) Social networking and mental health: looking beyond frequency of use and towards mechanisms of action. Neuropsychopharmacology 45:905–906

13. New York Times (2019) Human contact is now a luxury good. New York Times, March 23rd 2019. https://www.nytimes.com/2019/03/23/sunday-review/human-contact-luxury-screens.html. Accessed on May 13th 2020

14. Miner AS, Milstein A, Hancock JT (2017) Talking to machines about personal mental health problems. JAMA 318:1217–1218

15. Gratton L, Scott A (2016) The 100-year life. Bloomsbury, London

11

What Kind of Health Care System We Want

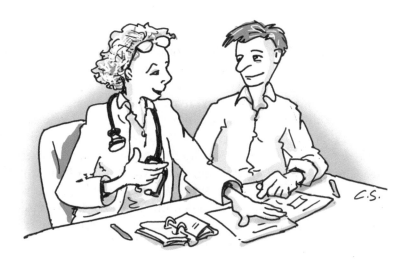

Abstract It is not the amount of money we invest in our health care system that determines our health. The US has by far the highest health care spending in the world, yet its life expectancy, which has actually been declining for several years, is mediocre by comparison, and Americans are among the most stressed and only moderately happy people. Significant social determinants of health are completely ignored by the American health care system. Governments that want to maintain and increase the health of a nation must reduce socioeconomic disparities, fight poverty, and provide the best possible education for all. A good health care system evolves from a primarily curative to a preventive system.

© Springer-Verlag GmbH Germany, part of Springer Nature 2022
G. Gründer, *How Do We Want to Live?*, https://doi.org/10.1007/978-3-662-64225-2_11

No country in the world spends more money per capita on health care than the US, and not by a long shot. The cost in the US is $9400, well over double the average of capitalist countries in the western world ($3600). The US spends 17% of its GDP on health care, a lone world leader [1]. In Germany in 2017, the share of health care spending was 11.5%, and the cost per capita was about 4500€. As recently as 2015, it had only been about 4000€, and less than 3000€ in 2005. Germany has the second highest health expenditure per capita in the EU after Luxembourg, and the highest share of GDP in this expenditure (EU average 9.9%). As everyone knows, despite their exorbitantly high health spending, US Americans are nevertheless no healthier than the rest of the world: life expectancy is higher in 39 countries than in the US, where it peaked at 78.8 years in 2014, only to fall slightly again since then (2017: 78.5 years). In 18 EU countries alone, life expectancy is higher than in the US, including Germany, where it is 81 years. The causes of these trends have been the subject of much of this book. The rising suicide figures in the USA were already a topic in Chap. 3. Even more explosive, however, is that between 1990 and 2017, drug overdose mortality increased by almost 400%. But there are other factors responsible for the fact that life expectancy in the US has plateaued for the past five years. Mortality rates among middle-aged people (25–64 years) due to obesity and hypertension increased by 114% and 79%, respectively, during this period, and mortality due to alcohol-associated diseases such as cirrhosis increased by 40% [2]. While the American press attributes these figures to the American lifestyle (especially lack of exercise and obesity, see Chap. 2) [3], Hans Rosling, whom we also heard about in Chap. 2, sees other major factors for the fact that American public health is in such a bad state despite the huge financial expenditures for the health care system: "The answer [to the question why US citizens cannot achieve the same level of health, and with the same expenditures, as other capitalist countries that have similar resources] is not difficult to find, by the way: It is because the U.S. lacks the kind of public health insurance that most citizens of other countries [...] take for granted. Under the current U.S. system, rich patients with private insurance see a doctor more often than they need to, while poor patients can't afford even simple, inexpensive treatments and die earlier than they should. Doctors waste time on unnecessary and pointless treatments that could be better spent saving lives or treating serious illnesses" [1].

Here, then, the question of the health care system—and even more: the entire political system—becomes decisive for the question of the health or illness of a people. Of course, even American scientists are fully aware that there are many social determinants of health. Where and under what conditions we are born and grow up is probably much more significant for our physical and especially mental health than any genes passed on to us by our parents. These conditions determine how we live, work and age. And it is also clear to American scientists that the lack of investment in social services and education, as well as a misguided medical care system, are responsible for the fact that despite the tremendous financial investment the American people make in their health, the results fall far short of what is possible [4]. It is also the responsibility of physicians to point out the importance of social conditions to the health of a nation, and they should use their influence and prestige to set policy. They must develop publicity for the fact that an individual patient's illness is influenced by factors beyond the control of the patient and the physician. A person who has a poor diet and whose illness is contributed to by that diet often cannot help the poverty which that diet causes.

In Chap. 7 I reported that today neuroscientists are trying to calculate a person's risk for a particular disease from their genetic risk profile, the so-called "polygenetic risk score". Something similar has now been proposed as a "polysocial risk score" [5]. If it makes sense to infer a person's risk of disease from their genetic profile, then it makes just as much sense for their social profile. The extent to which poverty or a lack of education, for example, are risk factors for disease, especially mental illness, I will elaborate in the next section. To contrast a polygenetic risk score with a polysocial risk score is an important step, because it expresses the fact that illness is not only caused by misguided individual biology, but also by the individual's position in the system. However, it is much less in keeping with the self-image of doctors to act prophylactically than curatively. Doctors usually take up their profession because they want to cure sick people or at least alleviate their suffering. It is undisputed that medicine has made tremendous progress in the treatment of most diseases. Our efforts to better understand the molecular processes involved in the development of disease must not be allowed to slacken. In the case of cancer, for example, who would not be grateful for the achievements of modern cancer therapy, which today usually enable a significant prolongation of life and often even a complete cure? For doctors, it is a special moment when they can discharge a patient home cured after a serious, often life-threatening illness, and for many this represents the essential—absolutely legitimate—motive for choosing this profession. We experience it much less as a reward to prevent the outbreak of a disease, that is, to take preventive action. Nevertheless, it is equally indisputable that it was not curative but primarily social medicine measures that led to the enormous increase in life expectancy over the last 100 years. Of course, it was first necessary to understand how infectious diseases spread through pathogens. But then it was primarily measures to improve hygiene, the monitoring of food and the systematic vaccination of entire populations that led to the drastic reduction in mortality from infectious diseases. Tuberculosis, plague and cholera no longer play a role anywhere in the world because we have practically eradicated them through hygienic measures. Prophylaxis through socio-medical measures was decisive here; we only take curative action (through the administration of antibiotics) when a flare-up of disease occurs somewhere in the world (for example, when natural disasters lead to the collapse of drinking water and sewage supplies and subsequently to an outbreak of cholera).

Curative medicine is also an economic factor with enormous economic significance. In Germany, one in eight employed people work in the health-care sector, which amounted to 5.6 million people in 2019 (Germany has about 45 million employed people). That's almost seven times as many people as are employed in the automotive industry (2019: 830,000 employed including all workers in the automotive supply industry), which likes to claim that it is Germany's most important industry. And even if the number of hospitals in Germany has been steadily declining for decades and is still far too high according to a report by the Bertelsmann Foundation, which caused a lot of discussion in 2019, hospitals still have a significant economic weight: in 2018, the statutory health insurance spent 77 billion € on hospital treatment in one of more than 1900 hospitals alone, and the value is steadily increasing by several percent annually. In 2000, the expenditure was still 44 billion €. Total health spending in Germany in 2017 was 376 billion € (for comparison, the 2020 federal budget was 362 billion € before a supplementary budget was passed due to the Corona crisis). For anyone benefiting from this system, further growth can only be desired. Hospital operators want 100% occupied beds, doctors want full surgeries, medical device manufacturers want to sell ever new, expensive (and no doubt ever better) devices, and pharmaceutical manufacturers want patients taking new, expensive, and not necessarily ever better drugs. For this reason, the healthcare sector is also a driver of innovation, because innovations promise billions in profits. Hundreds of biotech companies have sprung up in recent decades, dedicated to elucidating the molecular basis of all possible diseases and developing drugs that are tailor-made to target subtle dysfunctions underlying these diseases. Biotechnology, and drug development in particular, is a risky business. From the first idea, or the first molecule, to the market launch of a new drug usually takes more than ten years, time in which these companies burn many (hundreds of) millions of euros or dollars. Then, however, a single drug that is certified as effective and tolerable by the American or European regulatory authorities is enough to recoup the investment costs in many cases. I have already pointed out several times in this book that this business model has been extremely successful in cancer medicine in recent years. Nevertheless, it is estimated that 40% of all cancers could be prevented by lifestyle changes (e.g. avoiding obesity and lack of exercise, see Chap. 6), i.e. by simple and quite inexpensive prophylactic measures. However, we have also seen in Chap. 3 that the successes in psychopharmacology in the last 20 years have been modest in comparison, and I have already speculated on the reasons for this. The difficulties here lie in a fundamental lack of understanding of the relationship between brain function and psychological experience, and this in turn is determined not only by brain chemistry but also by the position of the individual in his social system. This also means, however, that the prophylaxis of mental illnesses must become much more of a focus, not only of psychiatry but also of politics, than it has been in the past. Here we need much more prophylactic—i.e. socio-medical—approaches, and this will also require completely new allocations of resources. Let no one misunderstand me: We need better therapies, and especially better effective and better tolerated medications for treating serious mental illness, and we need investment in that research. But if we want happier and more contented people who can develop creatively according to their potential and whose lives have meaning, then we will not achieve this by intervening in the brain to create the divine human being. And this fundamentally different understanding then also requires different, expanded approaches in a health care system.

References

1. Factfulness RH (2018) Wie wir lernen, die Welt so zu sehen, wie sie wirklich ist. Ullstein, Berlin
2. Woolf SH, Schoomaker H (2019) Life expectancy and mortality rates in the United States, 1959–2017. JAMA 322:1996–2016
3. CNN (2019) US life expectancy is still on the decline. Here's why. CNN, November 26th 2019. https://edition.cnn.com/2019/11/26/health/us-life-expectancy-decline-study/index.html. Accessed on May 14th 2020
4. Mani A, Mullainathan S, Shafir E, Thao J (2013) Poverty impedes cognitive function. Science 341:976–980
5. Figueroa JF, Frakt AB, Jha AK (2020) Addressing social determinants of health: time for a polysocial risk score. JAMA 323:1553–1554

12

How We Educate and Train

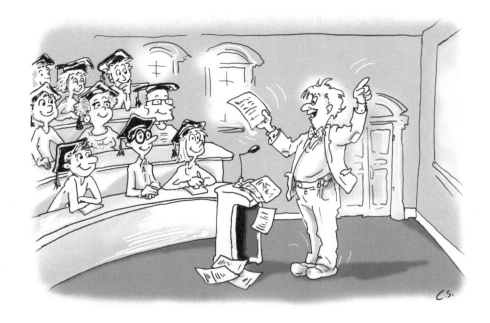

Abstract Poverty is an important determinant of mental health, and poverty is a consequence of a lack of education. We believe that intelligent, cognitively capable people achieve greater success, wealth and socio-economic status. However, this again expresses our biologistic-deterministic view of the world, according to which people are born with different, genetically determined abilities, and according to these abilities they achieve different levels of prosperity, wealth and status. However, it also works the other way around: poverty even affects our cognitive ability. Reduce poverty and people's cognitive performance increases, and so do their opportunities to shape their own lives. There is no better proven link than that between the risk of mental illness on the one hand and poverty and lack of education on the other. Education is an important key to better health.

We have already seen in Chap. 8 that lower social status is associated with higher stress, unhealthier nutrition and higher body weight [1]. Poverty is an extremely important determinant not only of physical health, but also of mental health (again, noting that this is only an artificial separation). We like to assume that intelligent, cognitively capable people make it to greater success, wealth, and socioeconomic status. However, this again expresses our biologistic deterministic worldview, according to which people are born with different genetically determined abilities, and according to these abilities they achieve different levels of wealth, prosperity and status. However, a British/US team of psychologists and economists has shown that the reverse can also be true: Poverty actually affects our cognitive performance.

We readily attribute unreasonable behaviors to people living in poverty: they are less health conscious and do not take advantage of health care offerings (e.g., preventive screenings), they do not keep appointments or do so unreliably, they work less productively, they are less attentive parents, and they manage their finances poorly. Not only are many of these behaviors problematic in their own right, they can further deepen poverty [2]. There are certainly a host of psychosocial factors that perpetuate this spiral. But poverty also appears to affect cognitive ability quite directly. Researchers tested this in two complementary studies. In the first, conducted in the laboratory, they tested the influence of (mental) preoccupation with financial challenges on cognitive performance in two groups of poorer and richer subjects. The 100 or so subjects were recruited from an American shopping mall. They represented a cross-section of socioeconomic conditions in the US. The subjects were presented with various scenarios such as the following, "Your car is having some trouble and requires $X to be fixed. You can pay in full, take a loan, or take a chance and forego the service at the moment... How would you go about making this decision?" They were then asked to think about the solution to this problem, imagining that it would trigger any existing worries of their own. They were then tested on their cognitive performance. There were two experimental conditions. In one condition ("easy"), the repair required only $150; in the second ("hard"), it cost $1500. It was suspected that facing significant financial burdens (in the "hard" condition) would be more likely to trigger one's own worries. Now, if you suspect that wealthy people are also more cognitively capable, you are mistaken. In the "easy" condition, the people with the low income were at most slightly, at least not statistically significantly, less efficient than the subjects with the high income. But in the "hard" condition, their performance fell very significantly behind that of the rich subjects.

The second study was a field experiment with nearly 500 farmers in India who grow sugarcane. Their socioeconomic status is highly seasonal. Before harvest, farmers typically live in poverty; after harvest, they have much more money. Before harvest, they are often in debt and have difficulty paying their bills. This time, the farmers were tested twice on their cognitive performance, once before and once after the harvest. In this experiment, too, the effect of financial worries on cognitive performance proved significant. In all tests, the farmers were significantly more efficient after the harvest [2].

How relevant are these effects in everyday life? To this end, it is interesting to look at how subjects' performance on exactly the same cognitive performance tests used in the experiments described here is affected by other factors. For example, the same magnitude of impairment as that caused by poverty is found after a full night's sleep deprivation. That is, if you go through a full night's sleep, you will be just as cognitively impaired as if you have to worry about your finances all the time. Or, perhaps to make it more vivid: The difference in cognitive performance between 60 year olds and 45 year olds is, on average, about the same as the difference in cognitive performance between the poor and the rich. Another example? People with chronic alcohol disease have about the same degree of cognitive impairment compared to healthy people as poor people compared to rich people. If you were to do an intelligence test, you would come up with a difference of about 13 IQ points [2].

Why am I presenting all this in such detail? Because, as the authors of the studies point out, these findings have important policy implications. They conclude that being poor does not simply mean coping with a lack of money, but also with a lack of cognitive resources. Poor people, they argue, are not less capable or successful simply because of their inherent (= innate!) characteristics, but because the context of poverty is a burden and impairs their cognitive abilities. In my view, however, the authors of the two studies then fail to reach the right, far-reaching conclusions. They call for policy to adjust its demands on poor people in terms of cognitive performance, just as low-income earners are asked to pay less or no taxes. They say that simple interventions need to be developed, such as simply structured forms or even automatic reminders, to adjust to lower cognitive resources. These would be the right measures if cognitive performance were indeed a purely biologically determined, inherent characteristic of an individual. Yet the study results show just that not! They show that when poverty is reduced, cognitive performance increases, and so do the opportunities to shape one's own life.

It has long been known that poverty is associated with poorer physical health. But this is equally true for mental health. People from poorer socio-economic backgrounds are significantly more likely to suffer from mental illness than people with higher or higher incomes. In Chap. 2, I referred to a study in which researchers from Finland investigated the influence of household income on the risk of being admitted to a psychiatric hospital for the first time. To do this, they had data for the entire Finnish population (just over 6.2 million people) living in Finland between 1996 and 2014. Like everywhere else in Western industrialized nations, both the number of psychiatric hospital beds and the length of stay have been steadily decreasing in recent decades. In the study now presented, a clear (negative) correlation was found between household income and the frequency of first-time psychiatric hospital treatment. The number of first-time treatments decreased with the level of household income. In addition, however, only people with the highest incomes were able to participate in the trend of decreasing psychiatric hospital beds. Among people with very low household incomes, an increase in first-time inpatient treatments was even registered in the first ten years of the observation period [3]. Now, one should not necessarily conclude from these figures that people with higher incomes are necessarily mentally healthier. They may use the health care system differently and seek outpatient services first. People with higher socioeconomic status are probably more able to adapt to new treatment modalities, as represented by the steady shift from inpatient to outpatient forms of care in recent decades. The correlation between household income and risk of first-time inpatient treatment may thus also say something about our health care system—conditions in Germany will not be fundamentally different from those in Finland. But that is certainly not the whole truth. Mental health itself is also unequally distributed, and this is particularly significant among young people. Many studies agree that the social environment is an important determinant of mental health, especially among young people. In Finland, the prevalence (frequency) of major depression among adolescents aged 14–16 years increased slightly overall in both sexes between 2000/2001 and 2010/2011. However, among adolescents whose parents were unemployed and had a low level of education, it almost doubled during these ten years, from 6.5% to 12.8% among boys and from 6.4% to 11.4% among girls [4]. Thus, boys were ten times and girls four times more likely to be affected by major depression than their peers from families with middle or high levels of education and whose parents were not affected by unemployment. These figures are also significant because, again, they are a reflection of the Finnish population as a whole. And they show an increase in mental health inequality as a function of the socioeconomic status of the population. Only recently, in March 2020, the answer of the Federal Government to a so-called "small inquiry" of the FDP parliamentary group about the "health opportunities of children and adolescents in Germany" went through the press in Germany. However, the answers were known beforehand, because already in the first sentence of its "question" the party states: "The health opportunities of children and adolescents in Germany are strongly dependent on the socio-cultural status of the parental home" [5]. The core statements can be summarized like this: Children from poorer families, which are primarily those in which neither parent is in full-time employment, have poorer health, they suffer more frequently from mental illnesses and developmental delays, they have a poorer diet and are more frequently overweight. For example, children from poorer socioeconomic backgrounds are 2.8–4.4 times more likely to suffer from attention deficit hyperactivity disorder (ADHD) than children from better-off homes. Traditionally, it would have been argued (and many still do) that children from poorer homes are more likely to suffer from ADHD because they have inherited the corresponding genes from their parents, and it is precisely these genes that have worsened educational opportunities in the parents' generation. But we have seen—and more examples will follow—that it is not that simple. The social milieu undoubtedly influences psychological well-being and cognitive performance.

In this context, the figures for the USA are interesting, where the socioeconomic differences are considerably greater than in any Scandinavian country and also greater than in Germany. I had already shown in Chap. 2 that the prevalence (remember: frequency related to a population group) of depression in the USA increased significantly from 2005 to 2015, and that this increase is not as rapid in any population group as it is among adolescents aged 12 to 17 [6]. And again, it is those with the lowest incomes and least education who are not only significantly more likely to be affected by depression than those with the highest socioeconomic status. Among them, moreover, the prevalences continue to rise. However, it is noticeable in the USA that people in the highest income groups and with the highest educational status are also affected by an increase in depression prevalences there, albeit at a much lower starting level than in the poorer population groups. Similar figures are available for many countries around the world, not just western industrialised nations, and there is arguably no better documented finding than the link between risk of mental illness on the one hand and poverty and lack of education on the other. It would be cynical to attribute these differences to common genetic causes and to claim that people with the "better" genes are just more intelligent, therefore have access to better education, consequently earn better, and are more resistant to mental stress because of these circumstances or again because of their "better" genes. The study above on the effect of poverty on cognitive performance is but a single piece of "academic" evidence that contradicts this. Quite different observations are even clearer: In Afghanistan, depression affects more than one in five people; the country has the highest prevalence of depression in the world [7]. But this is certainly not because Afghans have "worse" genes, but because of the poverty, insecurity and violence that have dominated this country for decades now. It is even more cynical—or simply ignorant—when Yuval Harari claims that the improvement of human living conditions is superseded by an intervention in the biochemistry of the brain, that this is the "path to happiness". This is exactly what the poor of the world try to do when they want to get a little break from their misery with a shot of heroin. That this is a path that only provides relief for hours or even minutes is well known.

But it will not be enough to reduce poverty in absolute, objective terms. We have seen in Chap. 2 that Hans Rosling in the last years before his death, especially with his book "Factfulness", tirelessly pointed out that living conditions on earth have steadily improved for more and more people. Rosling, for example, points out very clearly that in the last 20 years the proportion of the world's population living in extreme poverty has more than halved [8]. But this is only half the truth. What has not decreased in many countries of the world is the inequality of living conditions. Socio-economic disparities have increased rather than decreased. This is particularly impressive in the United States, where these differences are especially drastic and continue to increase. Only in Russia and India is wealth apparently more unequally distributed. According to recent data from the Federal Reserve, in 2019 the richest 1% of the American population owned about 32% of all the country's property, and the next richest 9% owned another 37%. That means the richest 10% of the population owns 69% of America's national wealth. In contrast, the entire poorer half (50%!) of the population owned only 1.6% of the wealth. Over the decades, this inequality has continued to grow. In 1989, the richest 1% of the population owned 24% of the wealth, while the poorer half still owned 3.7%. During and after the financial crisis, however, the gap had widened even further because the housing crisis had hit the middle class particularly hard [9]. If the total wealth of the American people were divided equally among all 62 million households, each household would have a fortune of an unfathomable $862,000! The reality, however, is that the poorer half of the population has household wealth averaging $11,000. This means that 50% of American households today have 50% less wealth on average, adjusted for inflation, than they did in 1989 [10].

In Germany, however, the situation is not fundamentally different. Germany is the country with the greatest inequality in the distribution of wealth in the euro area, and here, too, the inequality in the distribution of wealth is increasing. According to figures from 2007, the richest thousandth of the population owned 22.5% of total national wealth, the richest 1% owned 36% and the richest 10% owned 67%, while the poorer half of the population together owned 1.4% of total wealth [11]. So, by the standards by which Rosling measures poverty, the poorest people in the Western world may be much better off today than they were 20, 50 or 100 years ago. No one starves on the streets anymore. But the poorer people, be they the poorest 10%, 20% or even 30% are under at least as much pressure today as they were then, and it has probably even increased. Only a reduction in socio-economic disparities and an equalisation of living conditions would lead to a reduction in social stress in the poorer, less privileged sections of the population. Why is the richest country on earth, the United States, ranked only 19th in the United Nations' 2019 "World Happiness Report," just four places ahead of its much poorer southern neighbor, Mexico? [12]. In the first places are without exception the Scandinavian states, Finland ahead of Denmark, Norway, Iceland, in fifth place the Netherlands. All these states are distinguished by a social-democratic political system with a pronounced community system, which is concerned with social balance. Germany is only two places ahead of the USA in 17th place in the ranking. Interestingly, the problems that characterize the health—and especially the mental health—of the citizens of the United States, and which I have repeatedly addressed in this book, are explicitly discussed in the report as major causes of the dissatisfaction that prevails in the American population.

Why is satisfaction so relatively high in Mexico, and in Latin American countries in general, even though incomes there are so much lower than in the USA, and even though many citizens experience the country as extremely insecure? People in Mexico rate "personal relationships" as particularly positive, and it is precisely the quality of social relationships—the report emphasizes this in a separate chapter—that is of decisive importance for the quality of life of a country's citizens. Prosocial behavior, characterized above all by generosity, is a significant determinant of a person's well-being, but conversely, well-being also increases generous behavior. The authors write, "People are more likely to derive happiness from helping others when they feel free to choose whether or how to help, when they feel connected to the people they are helping, and when they can see how their help is making a difference." The report delivers a scathing verdict on the U.S. policy in an entire concluding chapter: "A variety of interrelated evolutionary, socioeconomic, physiological, and regulatory factors are associated with rising addiction rates across areas including drugs and alcohol, food and obesity, and internet usage. The United States' historical failure to implement public health policies that emphasize well-being over corporate interests must be addressed to respond to the addiction epidemic. Effective interventions might include a rapid scale-up of publicly financed mental health services and increased regulation of the prescriptive drug industry and other addictive products and activities" [12].

So improving socioeconomic conditions for as many people as possible, along with reducing those disparities, is the central key to better individual health and a healthier society, not brain intervention. And that path is through education. But what does good education look like? Should we teach our children to program computers and build robots as quickly and as comprehensively as possible? That seems to be the recipe for solving all of humanity's current problems, if you believe all those (and there are so many different professions, not just education politicians) who see salvation in more "digitalization". Germany (and if you are not a German citizen, replace "Germany" with your country, it won't be any different, unless you are US or Chinese) has lost touch in this field, and if our economy wants to still play a role in the future, we would have to invest in much more "digital education" today. But digititalization is only one aspect of technology as a major force shaping our future. As we saw in the section on the future of work, quite different forces are shaping our future, and we need to focus our attention on these too if we are to adapt our education system to these challenges.

The most important step is that really every child must have access to a good education, regardless of his or her background and the socio-economic status of his or her parents. Children's educational opportunities in Germany, and even more so in the USA, are still too dependent on their parents' education and income. The "Social Report for the Federal Republic of Germany", which is published every two years, showed again in 2018 that in Germany the social origin has a very strong influence on the later life of young people [13]. At high school (German: Gymnasium), two-thirds of students have parents with graduation from high school, but at secondary school (German: Hauptschule) only 16%. More than half of the pupils at secondary schools have parents who themselves have only a graduation from secondary school or no graduation at all. I have already pointed out above that children from homes with a lower socio-economic status are considerably more likely to have mental health problems. Children with a migration background, who are also at risk of poverty, must be considered particularly disadvantaged. Prevention of mental illness, depression, anxiety and addiction starts with education for the poor! Only good education, which is available to all, will prevent the emergence of a growing proletariat in Western countries (of course, this applies in principle to every country in the world, but I am writing here from an admittedly Western-centred perspective), which has no chance of earning its living in a globalised labour market over an increasingly long life span. In a world of work in which simpler jobs requiring fewer qualifications will in future be increasingly taken over by computers, machines and robots, it will be crucial that young people never stop learning and adapt flexibly to constantly changing living and working conditions.

Lynda Gratton argues that education must have the goal of enabling people to develop from shallow generalists who know a little bit about a lot to serial masters [14]. True mastery will be even more important in the future than it is today. A worker in production, for example on the assembly line in the car industry, has always been replaceable. In the future, however, there will be fewer and fewer such jobs. It will therefore be important in the future to create value for others or the community, and that value will be especially high the more masterful I am at my work and the fewer masters of my art are available. However, since it is highly likely that our world, and therefore the demands of the world of work, will continue to change rapidly in the future, it will be necessary to shift one's focus, to adapt, and to gain mastery in other, adjacent, and sometimes entirely different fields as well. It shows great naivety to now want to make our children fit for the challenges of the future by constantly proclaiming "digitalization". Who knows what role digitalization will play in 2050? For sure, our world will be so digitally organized that a large number of people will make a living from maintaining and further developing the digital infrastructure. But perhaps by then we will have identified completely different growth areas as drivers of innovation. Education must therefore, in my opinion, teach not so much topics as strategies. Children need to learn to be creative, to identify and solve problems, and to constantly adapt to new challenges. Lynda Gratton formulates five steps a learner should take today to prepare for the job market of the future (note: the word "digitilalization" does not appear in it) [14]:

- Try to understand *why* certain skills might be more valuable than others in the future.
- Try to anticipate *what* skills might be valued in the future.
- While you keep these skills and competencies in mind, do what you love!

- Then immerse yourself in this activity as deeply as possible to become a true master of your craft.
- Be prepared to adapt and develop mastery in other fields.

Gratton foresees that, at least in the next few decades, it will be social entrepreneurship and microentrepreneurship that will have a major impact on the work of many millions of people, although there will certainly be large multinational corporations in the future as well. What remains to be said is that this is not about teaching the "what?", i.e. what issues might be significant in the future, but about the "how?", i.e. how to deal with these issues creatively. If we create an education system that teaches these skills to our children—and to as many of them as possible—then we will have laid the foundations for happier and more contented next generations who will be able to tackle the major problems of the future.

References

1. Shively CA, Day SM (2014) Social inequalities in health in nonhuman primates. Neurobiol Stress 1:156–163
2. Mani A, Mullainathan S, Shafir E, Thao J (2013) Poverty impedes cognitive function. Science 341:976–980
3. Suokas K, Koivisto AM, Hakulinen C et al (2020) Association of income with the incidence rates of first psychiatric hospital admissions in Finland, 1996–2014. JAMA Psychiatry 77:274–284
4. Torikka A, Kaltial R, Rimpelä A, Sel et al (2000) to 2011. BMC Public Health 14:408
5. Kleine Anfrage der FDP-Fraktion an die Bundesregierung: "Gesundheitschancen von Kindern und Jugendlichen in Deutschland." https://dip21.bundestag.de/dip21/btd/19/173/1917385.pdf. Accessed on May 14th 2020
6. Weinberger AH, Gbedemah M, Martinez AM et al (2018) Trends in depression prevalence in the USA from 2005 to 2015: widening disparities in vulnerable groups. Psychol Med 48:1308–1315
7. Smith K (2014) Mental health: a world of depression. Nature 515:181
8. Factfulness RH (2018) Wie wir lernen, die Welt so zu sehen, wie sie wirklich ist. Ullstein, Berlin
9. Federal Reserve. Distribution of household wealth in the U.S. since 1989. Last Update December 23rd 2019 https://www.federalreserve.gov/releases/z1/dataviz/dfa/distribute/table/#quarter:120;series:Net%20worth;demographic:networth;population:all;units:shares. Accessed on May 14th 2020

10. Federal Reserve. Perspectives on inequality and opportunity from the survey of consumer finances. Speech by Chair Janet L. Yellen, October 17th 2014 https://www.federalreserve.gov/newsevents/speech/yellen20141017a.htm. Accessed on May 14th 2020
11. Bach S, Beznoska M, Steiner V. A wealth tax on the rich to bring down public debt? German Socio-Economic Panel Study, DIW Berlin. https://www.diw.de/documents/publikationen/73/diw_01.c.378111.de/diw_sp0397.pdf. Accessed on May 14th 2020
12. Helliwell JF, Layard R, Sachs JD World Happiness Report 2019. https://s3.amazonaws.com/happiness-report/2019/WHR19.pdf. Accessed on May 13th 2020
13. Wissenschaftszentrum Berlin für Sozialforschung. Datenreport 2018. Ein Sozialbericht für die Bundesrepublik Deutschland. https://www.wzb.eu/de/publikationen/datenreport/datenreport-2018. Accessed on May 14th 2020
14. Gratton L (2011) The shift. The future of work is already here. Harper Collins, London

13

Ways into the Future

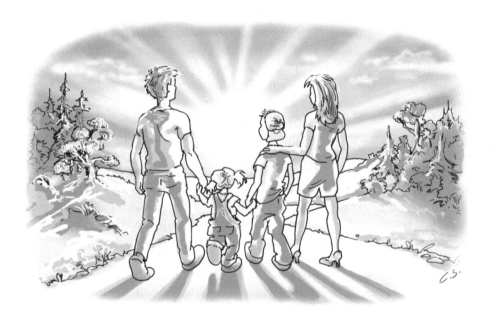

Abstract A better understanding of the biology of the brain has provided us with essential insights into human nature and the biological basis of mental illness. However, this alone will not be enough to address the 'global mental health crisis'. There are numerous socio-cultural factors that influence our wellbeing, and we can shape these ourselves. However, introducing a 15-hour working week or unconditional basic income will not fix the effects of poverty

G. Gründer, *How Do We Want to Live?*, https://doi.org/10.1007/978-3-662-64225-2_13

and inequality of wealth on our health. People won't get healthier by being given a bit more money for doing less or no work. They will need to educate and train themselves better to do work that fulfills them and makes them feel like they are making a meaningful contribution to the community and making life on this planet a little bit better, even if it's just in their smaller, local social network.

I wrote this book to counter the widespread biological reductionism in the life sciences. We will not be able to stem the enormous spread of mental illness by learning to understand the brain better and developing better drugs alone. We will need to do that, and it will help improve the treatment of these disorders. Many of my professional colleagues will take this book as a plea against the use of psychotropic drugs. But that is a gross misunderstanding, and anyone familiar with my work over the past 30 years will acknowledge that. Unquestionably, there are serious psychiatric illnesses that must be treated with psychotropic drugs. For many people, treatment with psychotropic drugs allows them back into a life in the community that they would not be able to have without one. Often that will have to be years of therapy, sometimes lifelong. But that alone will most certainly not be enough to address the "global mental health crisis." As good as much of his analysis is, in this respect Harari is most certainly barking up the wrong tree. I have presented a wealth of evidence for this in this book. The major epidemics of psychiatric illness do not originate in the brain—that is undoubtedly where they leave their mark— they originate in our society. One cannot attribute either the opioid crisis in the United States or the extreme prevalence of depression in Afghanistan to biological peculiarities of Americans or Afghans, respectively. There is simply no way around this without resorting to sociocultural explanations.

Why is this change of perspective important at all? If I consider my thinking, my feelings and all my actions as results of brain biochemical processes, then I deprive myself of my free will. Then the coexistence of human beings is determined by the interaction of many individual brains alone, and if the coexistence of human beings leads to the epidemic spread of depression, then the obvious conclusion is that I eliminate ("treat") the depression in those brains, for example by medication. This is how I then generate "global happiness" in Harari's sense. If, on the other hand, I perceive myself as an active agent in the interaction of human societies and consider happiness as the result of individuals living together in harmony, then I have an influence on how I feel. I go from being a passive bio-machine to being an active shaper of my future and the future of my living environment—and that of my children and grandchildren.

Will the 15-hour week or the unconditional basic income remedy the effects of poverty and the unequal distribution of wealth on our health, as the Dutch historian Rutger Bregman calls for in his bestseller "Utopia for Realists" [1]? Will it make people happier and more content if they don't have to work anymore, have even more free time and still get so much money from the state that they can live without existential angst, at least survive reasonably? I do not presume to judge the social appropriateness of Bregman's demands or their significance for our social systems. However, I do not believe that such an utopia makes people psychologically healthier—rather the opposite. I've laid out the reasons why. Many people will consume even more passively, for example watching TV, streaming series or playing video games, than they already do today, they will become bored and kill their time. Alcohol consumption will increase. I believe that improving living conditions and well-being for as many people as possible will not be achieved simply by redistributing wealth. Of course, wealth is more or less grotesquely unequally distributed in all societies, and the poor pay for it with poorer physical and mental health. But they will not get healthier by giving them a little more money for less or no work. They will have to be better educated and trained to do work that fulfils them and gives them the feeling that they are making a meaningful contribution to the community and making life on this planet a little bit better, even if it is only in the smaller, local social network. This education includes not only the transfer of knowledge ("digital literacy"!), but also playful problem-solving and thinking strategies and creativity. Above all, however, children, young people and even young adults must be made aware of the importance of real social interaction, which is not only conveyed via more or less small screens, because a meaning of one's own existence only arises in social interaction.

It may also sound a bit backward-looking in times when there are calls for more digital education to emphasize the importance of classical, humanistic education. By that I mean an education in history and especially philosophy. Man has asked himself the same questions at all times that have come down to us in some form: What am I living for? How should I live? What gives my life meaning and significance? How do I live my life in such a way that it feels right? How much material things does a person need? Is the pursuit of material goods perhaps even harmful? Do we need religion, spirituality? Despite all the industrialization, globalization, mechanization and digitalization, these questions are the same today as they were 2000 or 2500 years ago, and our answers seem to me no wiser today than they were then. Why are we witnessing such a remarkable renaissance of ancient philosophy, especially Stoicism and Epicureanism, in the life-skills literature in recent years? At the heart of these teachings was the proper conduct of life, the pursuit of bliss in a successful life, primarily through a balanced state of mind. We are no closer to that today, which was one of the central themes of this book, rather the opposite. While the questions have remained the same, we have not found satisfactory answers. The materialism that characterized the baby boomer generation has not made them any happier, and the generations that follow seem utterly disoriented in their constant, seemingly desperate search to keep up with their peers—but for some years now, not just in the same town or small city, but all over the planet (!). Dealing with these questions, whether in history, philosophy or religion classes, is part of training our children's minds if we don't believe that we can turn off feelings of meaninglessness, isolation and existential aloneness through Huxley's "soma" or Harari's more modern drugs—which we have yet to invent. Education, as I understand it, is education of the whole person, of body and mind as a unity, not the learning of some technique that is "in" at the moment but will be old news in twenty years at the latest.

Education for as many children and young people as possible also includes reducing poverty and reducing inequality in the distribution of wealth around the world. I have pointed out throughout this book, and provided ample evidence, that lack of education and poverty are among the most significant risk factors for mental disorders.

We will have to think about how we live and work together. This shows, particularly in the current Corona crisis, the enforced social isolation in which most people find themselves. I cannot understand how some of my professional colleagues can seriously think that the video conferencing model could replace face-to-face meetings in the future, because it has just been shown that virtual meetings also work well. Then one could also come up with the idea of moving the school completely to the Internet. Not only would we drastically reduce the risk of our children getting infected with germs and bringing them home. You wouldn't need any more school buildings (the good condition of which doesn't seem to be worth too much to us anyway), you would probably get by with considerably less staff, and the danger of accidents or even any arguments between pupils would be reduced. But what I said earlier about psychotherapy via video applies at least as much to scientific meetings, conferences, seminars, or even school teaching. In a pinch, it can all work for a while. But all these interactions between people are about much more than just the exchange of linguistic signals. People interact quite physically with each other, even when they are not touching. We don't talk about "body language" for nothing. Much of this cannot be conveyed via a computer screen. A good friend of mine, a psychiatrist in private practice, recently provided a nice illustration of this when he said that he already knew how a patient was feeling when he went with him from the waiting room to the consulting room without having exchanged a single word with him.

As humans, we are not just a brain in a body. We are always whole people interacting with others, our brain is just one—undoubtedly important—organ of interaction to exchange with other people and the nature around us. Reducing mental health to enabling our brain to function in a trouble-free molecular way is a reductionist aberration. It will not lead to greater well-being and serenity. Rather, as humans, we are part of nature and thus connected to it and embedded in it. We have seen that health and well-being require a minimum of connection with nature, and we will have to design our living environment accordingly. Only in cities that offer the most extensive green spaces possible will we feel healthy and well. At the same time, these cities must provide spaces for social interaction. As the world's population continues to rise in this century, these requirements will pose particular challenges for urban planners in the megacities of Asia and Africa. By designing our cities in a green way that not only facilitates genuine social interaction but also encourages it, we will be able to reduce the burden of mental illness on many millions of people, and ultimately on countries and national budgets. Therapy for a billion people, with a steadily rising trend especially in the still developing world, cannot be the solution.

I have also devoted a whole chapter to the question of how we want to work together in the future. It will certainly not make us healthier and certainly not happier people if we do more and more of our professional communication only through computer screens and are exposed to a permanent information bombardment through email and social media. We will have to work in smaller, more manageable social networks with real "physical" contacts. This is not incompatible with globalized communication in an international network, it just needs to be put into a reasonable and, above all, healthy relationship. We need to relearn that multitasking is not only ineffective, but also robs us of our cognitive abilities and makes us sick in the long run. Most of us spend such a tremendous amount of our lives working that it must be of particular concern to each of us to be equally constantly evolving in an ever-changing world. We must teach our children that learning and education are not a temporary, early phase of our lives, but must be a way of life.

All of the above approaches are ultimately prophylactic measures to help us maintain our physical and mental health for as long as possible. It is predominantly political measures, not medical ones, that are called for here. This requires us psychiatrists to become more political. Since the beginning of my professional career—and almost certainly before—psychiatrists who rely on the healing power of psychotropic drugs have waged a constant war of faith against psychotherapists (usually psychologists who do not have the ability to prescribe drugs) over the best and most effective therapy. Psychiatrists who are self-critical of the uncritical prescribing of psychotropic drugs are accused by their peers of "fouling their nests" and of wanting to abolish their own discipline. The debate about the biological versus social ("nature" versus "nurture") conditionality of mental disorders is just as bitter. An argument about an either/or is, however, devoid of content. In this book I have shown that it neither makes sense nor can lead to the goal of trying to adapt people to an environment that no longer corresponds to their nature by means of a purposeful intervention in brain chemistry. I don't even want to talk about the claim to make them happier or even healthier beings in the process. I have provided countless proofs that we can reduce psychological suffering at least as much by shaping our living environment as by any form of therapy, be it biological or psychotherapeutic. Nevertheless, psychiatric illness will always exist, even if we create optimal living conditions for all people on this earth. An optimal social environment for achieving the greatest possible mental health is as much an illusion as an optimal brain chemistry environment. The human mind is not deterministic, and as long as it will go in search of its destiny every day, it will experience failures, aberrations and crises, and sometimes even fail.

Reference

1. Bregman R (2017) Utopia for realists. Bloomsbury Publishing, London

Index

© Springer-Verlag GmbH Germany, part of Springer Nature 2022
G. Gründer, *How Do We Want to Live?*, https://doi.org/10.1007/978-3-662-64225-2